"A fine and heartfelt memoir from an author hopeful in his determination to endure against the odds: 'What remains is desire.'" —*Kirkus Reviews*

"Darkly funny and emotional, Fitzmaurice's story is as inspirational as memoirs get—he even wrote the entire book with an eye-gaze computer. This is a true story about family, health, and the true meaning of life that you won't want to miss." —*BookTrib*

"Daringly, brutally poignant, *It's Not Yet Dark* is the closest thing to pure love that I have read since *The Shack* and just as memorable . . . Like an Irish mist, *It's Not Yet Dark* unveils all pretense of living with an illness that kills daily, that can terminate life at any moment, leaving the brilliance and elegance of a writer at his best, peeling his life like an onion, living with presence and love at every opportunity. Thrillingly, achingly authentic prose that reveals an inner life of one human being with the courage to live fully every single moment of his life. Compromised as it is, Simon Fitzmaurice's life is a complete and miraculous act of loving life."
—*The Review Broads*

"A fierce, tender, and compelling examination of what it means to live." —*Brooklyn Bugle*

It's Not Yet Dark

It's Not Yet Dark

SIMON FITZMAURICE

Mariner Books
Houghton Mifflin Harcourt
Boston New York

First Mariner Books edition 2018

hmhco.com

First published in Ireland in 2014 by Hachette Books Ireland

Library of Congress Cataloging-in-Publication Data
Names: Fitzmaurice, Simon, author.
Title: It's not yet dark : a memoir / Simon Fitzmaurice.
Description: Boston : Houghton Mifflin Harcourt, 2017.
Identifiers: LCCN 2017027387 (print) |
LCCN 2017016109 (ebook) | ISBN 9781328918581
(ebook) | ISBN 9781328916716 (hardback) |
ISBN 9781328508270 (paperback.)
Subjects: LCSH: Fitzmaurice, Simon. |
Fitzmaurice, Simon—Health. |
Amyotrophic lateral sclerosis. | BISAC: BIOGRAPHY &
AUTOBIOGRAPHY / Personal Memoirs. | BIOGRAPHY &
AUTOBIOGRAPHY / Medical. | BIOGRAPHY & AUTOBIOGRAPHY
/ Entertainment & Performing Arts. | HEALTH &
FITNESS / Diseases / Nervous System (incl. Brain).
Classification: LCC RC406.A24 (print) | LCC RC406.
A24 F58 2017 (ebook) | DDC 616.8/39—dc23
LC record available at https://lccn.loc.gov/2017027387

Printed in the United States of America
DOC 10 9 8 7 6 5 4 3 2 1

For Ruth,
Jack, Raife, Arden, Sadie and Hunter

The brave

I am a stranger. A different breed. I move among you but am so different that to pretend I am the same only causes me pain. And yet I am the same, in as many ways as I am different. I am a stranger.

I observe your meaning on television, through song and writing. I was once like you. But I often feel distant from you.

My meaning has faces, names. Totems. The words we utter. Every breath of us is meaning.

Everyone notices but no one sees.

On the streets, in the crowds, no one sees.

I was once invisible. I moved among you, invisible in my disguise. Now I am difference made manifest. I cannot hide. I move with a force field that makes you avert your eyes. Only children see me. You gather them together when I draw near but they do not look away. You cross the street from me but your children do not look away. They are still looking for the definition of man.

I frighten you. I am a totem of fear. Sickness, madness, death. I am a touchstone to be avoided.

But not by all. The brave approach. Women. Children. Some rare men. And I am shaken awake.

Those I count as friends are the brave.

Holding my breath

I'm driving through the English countryside. A narrow road rising up to a tall oak tree. It could be Ireland. The call comes just before I reach the tree. It's my producer and she is excited. She has just received a call from the Sundance Film Festival, saying they would like to screen our film. I feel something shift inside me. She talks quickly, then gets off. I pass the tree. She calls back. Says she got another call and that they are really excited to screen our film. We exchange words of jubilation I can't remember and say goodbye. I'm driving down the country road and I am changed.

I have been to many other festivals. I don't know why this one means so much to me. Maybe it's because I grew up within my father's world of cinema, where Robert Redford was a legend. *The Natural* was one of our favourite films. I don't know. But I've often wondered if that was the moment motor neurone disease, or amyotrophic lateral sclerosis (ALS), began in me. That I had been holding my breath for years. And suddenly let go. And that something gave in that moment. Something gave.

My foot drops the following month.

I'm walking through Dublin. From Rialto to Stephen's Green. I stayed in a friend's house the night before. Slept on the floor. Now I hear a slapping sound. My foot on the pavement.

It's a strange thing, like my foot has gone to sleep and is limp. It passes. I immediately relate it to the shoes I'm wearing, brown and red funky things with no support whatsoever. I wonder if I damaged my foot on the mountain climb last year. So I go into the outdoors shop off Grafton

Street, upstairs to the footwear department, and start trying on a pair of running shoes, determined to give my foot support.

I ask the salesman for assistance. This is a mountaineering shop so I feel confident he will understand and I start to explain how I'd climbed a Himalayan mountain last year but I'd been wearing these awful shoes with no support and now my foot has started to flop in them and had he ever seen something like that before? He looks at me. My innocence meets his concern. No, I've never seen anything like that before, he says. The look in his eyes becomes a twinge in my stomach.

My first diagnosis is by a shoe salesman.

Baggot Street Bridge

I'm sitting on an uncomfortable stool in the dingy basement apartment of a friend from college when a girl walks into the room. She is tall, slender and quite easily the most beautiful girl I have ever seen. She is crossing the back of the room with a friend of mine. My first thought is simply, How the hell did he get her? She is a girl from Ardee, County Louth. She is out of my league. Her name is Ruth.

I spent my whole life looking for Ruth.

Years after first seeing her, I'm walking down O'Connell Street with my parents, after coming out of the Savoy cinema, and I pass Ruth at a bus stop outside Clery's department store. I stop my parents and run back to her. We talk but behind our words, in our eyes meeting, something is there. I ask for her number and she opens her bag. Her hair is short and she looks stunning in a simple navy winter coat. I'm cheeky. I see her pay slip in her bag and reach in, pretending to have a look. Ruth gives me her number, we say goodbye and I catch up with my parents. It's Thursday.

I don't call. It's too important.

The following Monday, I'm walking up from Lansdowne station into work. Coming back from working in Ukraine, I had got a job no one else wanted. It was an accountancy practice with one accountant. That was the staff. Me and him. My job was to sit in a little back office and answer the phone. It never rang. Ever. I read all day. It was so quiet that the recruitment agency said no one had lasted more than a week in the place before me. I was getting through a book every three days. Paid to read. I had been there for months.

I'm standing at Baggot Street Bridge, waiting to cross in a crowd of commuters. It's pre-coffee early and I'm half asleep. The girl in front of me is wearing headphones. Her coat is navy. I realise and slowly reach out to touch her shoulder. Ruth turns around. She is half asleep and it takes her a moment to recognise me. She goes red. I go red. She fumbles off her headphones and the crowd crosses the bridge without us.

It takes a few moments of conversation to figure out that she works just down the road from me and has done for months. That we both walk the same way to work, at the same time, and have done for months. But that we hadn't met until four days after we bumped into each other for the first time in years. Wonderfully weird.

Embarrassed beyond reason, we hurry off.

We meet for lunch in Searson's pub on Baggot Street. Two large bowls of pasta sit between us. But my stomach is constricted. So is Ruth's. We cannot eat. It is embarrassing. It is love.

At the weekend we go to the cinema with some friends. I sit beside Ruth. The air is magnetically charged with my desire to touch her.

We kiss for the first time a week after, in a basement nightclub off Wicklow Street, in the shadow of a doorway.

Empire State Building

This is it. My life is changed for ever.

My family is used to me talking all about love and the new person in my life. This time I tell them nothing. I let them meet Ruth for themselves. They are all nervous because of it. Ruth arrives and I watch her talk, move, blush and sit among them. I've never felt prouder in my life.

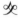

Ruth. My whole body is on fire. I've been in love before but never like this. It is not one thing or a list of things. It is everything. I'm in a different place than I've ever been. This is beyond any happiness I've felt. It's not what we do or say, it's about being together. It's wordless. We are animals, humans without words. I spend three days in her room. We only come out to eat. Sit in the back of taxis and travel wordlessly into Dublin to eat. We are creating a bond for life. It's obvious. We are consuming each other.

I have never felt more alive with anyone or been with anyone more alive. This is it.

I saved every penny, enough to put a deposit on a tiny three-bedroom mid-terrace railway cottage in the old part of Inchicore in Dublin. I buy it, rent out two bedrooms to friends to help pay the mortgage, and move in.

After a few months, Ruth moves in. She has just started working at Today FM, a national radio station, and is loving it. Broadcasting is her passion.

I do a web-design course for the sole reason that they have a digital video module. I direct three short films. No budget, shot on digital.

With Ruth I feel like I can do anything. I decide to do one last year of university to pursue my dream. I start a master's degree in film theory and production at the Dublin Institute of Technology. I get a job as a waiter in a pizza restaurant on the quays of the river Liffey.

Ruth and I are inseparable. She is unlike anyone else. We drive around in my little white car — her father calls it the Molecule. I meet Ruth's family. She has four brothers and a sister. Four. I'm nervous as hell. Ruth laughs as I stop the car at a crossroads before her house and change my shoes. A pair of black shiny ones I never wear. Her family is like my own. Close. Crazy. Boisterous in talk around the table. Full of love and humour, good food and wine. My kind of people.

Ruth and I eat in restaurants all around Dublin. We quickly find our favourites. We adore good food together. I don't know what we talk about. It's not important. We laugh at the same things. We devour narrative, books and films. We talk about that, I expect. I'm too busy looking at Ruth to remember.

We are happy and alive in the light from our bedroom window.

The film school has film cameras. Film-editing tables. Lights. Sound equipment. And a teaching staff committed to and passionate about film. I'm in heaven.

I write and direct a five-minute film. Shot on film, not digital, with a properly organised crew. Standing on set, walking among the cables and the beautiful chaos of people, all working towards a single creative purpose, I just feel right. This is what I want to do with my working life. I'm hooked.

Ruth is promoted at work. She is now producer of the afternoon show.

I write a simple love story about a girl who works in a chip shop and a guy who is a security guard at the bank across the road. They watch each other from a distance, neither of them knowing. It's my graduation film, fifteen minutes long, and I work on it night and day for a year. I graduate with first-class honours and a finished film, *Full Circle*, in my pocket.

The course is over and the students go their separate ways. I start sending my film out to festivals, three submissions a week. I get a job through my brother-in-law, Chris, at an asset-management company. It's data entry, monkey work, but it pays better than waiting tables. It's three days a week and a woman there takes pleasure in giving me the most menial jobs.

My film gets selected for the Cork Film Festival. It's screening on a Thursday and everyone involved is working so I ask my mum and we travel down by train, the two of us. Spending time with Mum is effortless. It's my first film festival and we sit in the dark and watch my film among the audience. It's magical.

Afterwards we get the train back to Dublin.

The call comes on Sunday morning. Ruth and I are asleep and the phone wakes me. It's someone telling me my film has won the Cork Film Festival. You're taking the piss, I say. Laughter on the phone. No, the voice says.

Ruth and I just make the train, sprinting down the platform. A few hours later, I'm standing back stage at the festival about to go on. A guy whispers in my ear. You see the awards? he says. I see a table of them on stage. I nod. That's your one, he says, the big one at the back.

I see it. They call my name.

I get a director's job in Chicago, a corporate project for a giant pharmaceutical company, bizarre in-house mumbo-jumbo. I don't care. I'm directing camera, crew and actors, in the smell of Chicago. I get up every day and go running before dawn in the city streets.

At my data-entry job I suggest to one of the directors that their website could do with a revamp and show him my ideas. Do it, he says. Within a year, I'm working full time, in charge of all the company's advertising, print, radio, online and TV. I give an advertising update at the weekly company meeting. I catch the eye of the woman who enjoyed giving me the shit detail. We don't have much contact any more.

❧

I drive up to Ardee, County Louth. I'm going to ask Ruth's parents for their permission to ask Ruth to marry me. I'm very specific about it. I'm not asking for their permission to marry Ruth. I'm asking for their permission *to ask Ruth*. It's my modern version of the old tradition. It's the way I was brought up, to respect parents.

I turn off the motorway, drive down the country road and come to the crossroads. I stop. Left is the road to Ruth's parents. Right is a road I've never taken before.

I'm going to ask Ruth's parents whether I can ask their daughter if she will marry me. Forever. For the rest of my life. I'm terrified. I take the road to the right.

Without purpose, without reason, I drive down the wrong road. I'm driving away from decision, from commitment. The road turns and reveals a row of poplar trees on the left-hand side. I've never seen poplar trees in Ireland. A wall of green, shivering in the wind. I drive down the length of them, fast. What am I doing? I reach the end and turn around, racing back down the row of swaying trees. Back to the crossroads.

I stop, open the door and sit my feet into the road. There is no one around. Not a soul.

A dog appears. A little terrier. He trots up the road and stops in front of me. Our eyes meet. Neither of us looks away. My mind is made up. I close the door and drive down the other road.

Full Circle is invited to screen at the legendary NYU Film School, so Ruth and I go to New York. The city steals our hearts. It's everything. The smell of the city. The deli next door to the hotel, open all night, with the most delicious salad bar we've ever encountered. We often just fill the plastic boxes and bring the food up to our hotel room for dinner, the window open to the sound of taxi horns as the lights brighten in the darkness.

I have never been more nervous. It's on my mind all the time and Ruth doesn't have a clue.

We're doing all this film stuff, meet-and-greets and screenings. We're visiting the Statue of Liberty and all the time I'm thinking, How will I do this? When? When?

I decide.

I phone the number my American cousin gave me, of friends of his living in New York City. I tell them my plan and ask for a recommendation for a restaurant after I ask Ruth. I book it.

At the end of the NYU screening of films, a man stands up and says that the overriding theme of the films was the uncomfortableness of being alive, and Ruth and I look at each other. We, and my little film about love, don't fit in there.

The next day, we visit the Empire State Building. This is where I'm going to do it. It's hot, really hot, yet I'm wearing my big jacket to hide the snipe of champagne and two *I love New York* shot glasses. I was nearly caught buying both but got away with it. Inside there is a queue for the elevators to the top. I'm sweating. Why don't you take off your coat? Ruth says. I'm ok, I say. I feel sick.

We turn a corner in the queue. People are lining up before a metal detector, putting their bags through an X-ray machine. Oh, shit. If they make me take off my coat the bottle will clink or show up on the screen and Ruth will know for sure. If she doesn't know already from my odd behaviour. God, I'm so hot. Sweat is running down my face. We approach the machine and the guards. I feel like a terrorist. Ruth puts her bag on the belt and goes through. They are going to stop me and ruin everything. They don't. We are in the lift. I smile at Ruth, sweat down the back of my neck. She must think I'm crazy.

At the top of the Empire State Building, as green as Kermit the frog, and with a similar voice, I get down on one knee and ask Ruth to marry me and she says yes.

I say his name

Ruth said yes. We are married. I sell Inchicore and we buy a little house in Greystones, the coastal town in County Wicklow where I grew up. We make it our own. My uncle Tony builds us simple bookshelves for all our books. Our first home.

Nine months later Jack is born. Our first born.

Back in the ward, Ruth and I look at our sleeping son. Ruth says she has a headache. It quickly escalates. She starts getting sick. Doctors come. Two of them stand at the end of the bed as Ruth is moaning in pain. They are discussing whether Ruth should have a cup of tea or maybe some paracetamol. I'm incredulous. Ruth starts screaming. Nurses come running. Ruth grips my hand and is saying my name over and over. Simon, make it stop. Simon, make it stop. I shout at them to give Ruth something for the pain. Ruth is crying. The doctor says they can't mask the pain, it is most likely a reaction to the epidural but they have to rule out a blood clot with an MRI. The ambulance is here, a nurse says. What? I say. Another nurse steps up to me, speaks quietly in my ear. There is a problem with your baby's breathing, we have to take him up to intensive care, she says. What? I say. Everything is spinning. I see Mum in the doorway, flowers in her hand, smiling. Jesus, Mum, you go with Jack, stay with him, I say, as I go out the door with Ruth to the ambulance.

Ruth is delirious with the pain, drenched in sweat, mumbling my name as we fly across the city, sirens blaring.

I stand outside the room as Ruth is being

scanned. The ambulance staff wait with me. They are not afraid of looking me in the eye. In the worst moments of my life.

Ruth is declared ok and they drive us back in silence across the city. The doctors give Ruth something and she is instantly asleep. I go up and Jack is ok. He is so big he barely fits into the incubator. He is back down beside Ruth the following day. They are ok.

Ruth quits Today FM to be with Jack.

I go running on the cliff walk just down from our house.

When Jack is a little older I walk him down and hold him up to see the trains. He is a wonder.

I'm full time in the advertising position while working on my films every spare minute. I'm travelling to film festivals with *Full Circle* and working on my new film, *The Sound of People*. It's a film about a moment in the life of an eighteen-year-old boy in which he confronts his mortality, and the mental and emotional journey it takes him on in a matter of seconds. It's intense. It started when I wrote on a piece of paper, 'The day after I die there will be internet.' The story grew out of that line. I wanted to make something different from the standard narrative structure. I wanted stream-of-consciousness on film.

Raife is born.

No epidural. No headache.

I wheel him down the corridor in his cot to be weighed, while Ruth sleeps. I watch him sleeping, breathing. I say his name like an incantation. Raife. Soft, gentle soul.

I finish *The Sound of People.* Ruth and I decide to leave Greystones to focus fully on our passions of film and writing. We sell our house. We make a plan.

The Sound of People is selected for the Sundance Film Festival.

After spending the night at a friend's house in Rialto, I'm walking into Dublin city centre. I hear a strange slapping sound. It's my foot on the pavement.

North Cottage

He meets us at the gate, holds it open, beckons us in. We drive across the frozen white gravel, crunching to a halt. The estate agent takes us inside. It's as if the owners have just stepped out. There is a roaring fire in the sitting room, a picture-perfect Christmas tree in the corner. It's a two-hundred-year-old cottage, lovingly restored in every aspect. Ruth and I walk from room to room in the utter silence that can mean only one thing. This is it.

I spend my days painting. We're living with Ruth's parents while we get the place ready.

So I'm here by myself while Ruth minds our children at her mum's.

There is no way better to get to know a house than to paint it. Down on your hands and knees in every corner of every room, a house reveals itself to you.

This house, this house we bought, is on the border of Louth and Monaghan. There are no neighbours either side, just fields in every direction, stretching to the horizon. We have almost an acre. Eight little apple trees standing in two rows. Strawberries from an overgrown herb garden. And a separate building, a garage, with a loft. There are two entrances. New wooden gates with a gravel driveway and, at the far side of the cottage, the original stone gateposts, lichened and mottled with time.

The trees that shadow the cottage sough in the breeze, and behind the hedgerow, the soft muffled hoof-falls of dray horses.

I'm standing in the cool interior of the garage. This is what drew me here, to be honest, this space. It is two-thirds the size of our previous house. A blank canvas of bare concrete walls. A window looking out into the garden. Perfect place for a desk. I have a vision. Home office. Home cinema. Turn the loft into a bedroom for visitors. Put a bathroom down here. Turn this concrete shell into a studio.

I'm painting the bathroom in the cottage. The ceiling. My arms feel funny. Like it's hard to hold them up there. It passes. I stand in the bedroom, the double doors open to the garden. I've finished painting the house. There is no sound but the movement of the wind, and the fields stretch out to an open sky. We move in and call it North Cottage.

Sundance

It never snows here, not ever. He said he'd lived in Atlanta for thirty years. I mean, I've seen sleet and hail, he said, staring out of the airport window, but not this fluffy floating stuff. Panic in Atlanta: snow.

Travelling and doing the numbers. Eight hours transatlantic. And then? Five more to Salt Lake City. Which time zone? How many hours ahead, behind? Start pretending you're on local time.

Descending into Atlanta I get excited for the first time about Sundance. Only another flight away. Out of the oval window, light snow is falling, like the beginning of something. And yet. Snow in Atlanta?

We get on the connecting flight and everyone is talking about the weather. Unlocking the bathroom door, the light dims and it feels like Christmas. A group of young men wearing similar suits and ties sit together like a team. They wear badges with the words *Jesu Christos* beneath their names: *Elder Jepson*; *Elder Koons*. None of them out of their early twenties. Some younger. They're a lively bunch, laughing and joking. Going home.

We taxi out from the terminal and come to a stop. It's still snowing. The captain tells us each plane has to be de-iced and describes the procedure. It's complicated and involves the wings and wheels. We're not used to this here in Atlanta, he tells us, so it may take a little while. Panic in the air: snow. After an hour of sitting on the tarmac, the captain explains we are in a queue for the de-icer and it's a line of ten planes. We're number ten.

Hours pass. The captain keeps a tally of our position in the queue. Seventh place. Children start to run in the aisles. Sixth. A man opposite shouts at an airhostess. Fourth. Two men break out a dominoes board and play across the aisle.

Second. A woman is crying, saying something about her daughter. A sleeping boy's feet stick out into the aisle. We've been in the plane for seven hours. First place: people cheer. We start to move. The captain comes over the intercom. I'm afraid I've got some bad news, folks, he says. Silence. Our duty shift has run out and I'm afraid we have to go back to the terminal. Silence. People are too stunned to even complain. It's inconceivable. The plane turns back.

Parents carry sleeping children from the plane. It's two in the morning. The terminal is like a refugee camp. Hundreds of people stranded. The largest queue I've ever seen snakes back and forth towards an airline desk. Two girls sit behind it. I ask around. Nobody knows what the queue is for, whether for re-booking flights or hotels or just information. I walk to the top and ask one of the women the purpose of the queue. She refuses to answer, saying I have to get in line. But if you'll just tell me what the line is for, I say. I'm sorry, sir, you'll have to get in line.

I persist. She calls the police. On her walkie-talkie. You can see them coming a mile off. Four of them. Badges, guns. I melt back into the crowd.

The airline makes an announcement: all hotels in the Atlanta area are booked out. We lie all night on the tile floor of the airport. Children sleep with their heads on their parents' laps. Elderly couples sit staring, unable to sleep. Hundreds of people fill the corridors, curled up with their bags for pillows. The tiles are cold.

In the morning I walk back to the main atrium and people are asleep in piles on the floor, the remnant of the massive queue, afraid to lose their place. The airline makes another announcement, stating that transatlantic passengers have been automatically reassigned places on the next available flights. We leave Atlanta.

Main Street, Park City, Utah. Night in Sundance. The crowd is heaving. Cameras point across the street. Every angle filled with fellow cameramen pointing back. The will to capture: the moment. Celebrities. Free merchandising. Main Street, Sundance, is a baptism of fire. Like a bus ride through downtown Delhi at night or – as a passer-by put it – a nuclear winter in Mardi Gras. It's snowing – the fluffy stuff – and the altitude shortens your frosting breath. The streets are humpbacked with snow, and between the buildings – in the darkness beyond Main Street – are mountains of impossible beauty.

The crowds are alive with anticipation. Hunger. An almost tangible will to consume the fame they know is hiding in expensive restaurants all around them.

Adoration has always been a troubling concept for me. Screaming crowds at rock concerts. The suspicion that fame is the will to defer responsibility to another. *The king is dead, long live the king.* That kind of thing. Sundance forces you to reflect on fame and art.

At the top of Main Street, at the peak of the madness, I pass a basement place called The Music Café and go down. It is packed and a woman is singing. All the lights are out but for the stage and we sit there in the dark, listening. She puts me in my place. Shuts me up and makes me sit there, listening as hard as I can. I realise it's not adoration when you find yourself listening to someone that way. It's inspiration. It's why we sit in the dark in cinemas or scream at concerts. It's exultation.

Robert Redford said he set up Sundance in the mountain town of Park City so it would be 'a little bit difficult to get to and a bit weird'. The snow in Atlanta ensured the former and, as for the latter, as a summit retreat for weirdness, it's alive and well.

Its mountaintop location doesn't hold off the marketing mania but Sundance is about people who love films. Whether you're a believer or not is down to your opinion. Just like an opinion on a particular film. The films I saw knocked me down and picked me up. So I'm a believer.

I had no expectations coming over here. All I knew was an idea of Sundance, like everybody else. I've seen dramas and documentaries here that have moved and pushed me, and because I'm here with a film, I'm forced to question whether my short film would move anyone that way. Scary.

In the morning I'm invited up to Robert Redford's house in the mountains.

No media, no producers, only directors. We travel up by coach, every director in the festival. The house is the soft colour of wood, with towering windows that let in the vast whiteness outside. There is a buffet laid on and it is sumptuous. After we've eaten, Robert comes out to greet us. He talks to us about the festival, what it means to him, the importance of film and directing to him. I'm listening and not listening, drinking in the brightness of the room. Afterwards I meet him and we talk about Dublin, people all around us. I meet Quentin Tarantino and he talks staccato. I give him a copy of my film and he puts it on top of a large pile on the table beside him.

I climb the street humped high with snow. I'm wearing boots and the snow is falling heavy and thick. I've just come from a screening of my film at the Egyptian Theater on Main Street. And I'm electrified. I decide to walk, out of the town, into the snow. There are other shops out here and I want to buy some presents for home. I walk along the edge of a larger road, the blizzard really picking up now. I love it here. I feel like a filmmaker for the first time in all my years dreaming about film. I reach the shops at the end of town. I step under a walkway and call my parents' house. My mother answers and I listen to her voice as I watch the cars pass slowly on the road through the blizzard. I tell her my foot is hurting, that there's something wrong with my foot. But we talk about it normally, neither of us is worried. Afterwards I head back towards town.

That night I go to a party in a mountain lodge. When it's late I go outside onto the balcony for a cigarette (don't tell my wife). There is a full moon and the mountains are cast in a blue light that makes the snow iridescent. It is something I have never seen.

Pain

Ruth has a miscarriage. It devastates us both.

It is a strange time for me. My foot is constantly on my mind. I'm seeing a neurologist for tests.

The day after the miscarriage I'm driving from North Cottage to Dublin for a nerve test called an EMG (electromyogram). We are already under a lot of pressure, worry, stress.

I'm on the M1 in the car by myself and I'm angry at the pain I saw the miscarriage causing Ruth.

I don't think I've ever felt so angry.

And yet I feel detached from it, feel nothing,

and that doubles my anger and shame at myself for such feelings.

And I say something.

I say, I hope this hurts.

I hope this procedure I'm about to undergo hurts me.

Because I want to be hurt. For Ruth, for me, for this loss that we've suffered.

I say it out into the world, throw it through my teeth at the clouds.

It was a mistake.

The procedure turned out to be the most pain I have ever experienced.

Someone heard me.

It has been said that it's impossible to remember pain.

I will never not remember this.

He sticks long needles directly into my nerves. Like that moment a dentist accidentally touches a nerve. Except this is deliberate, and he doesn't just touch it, he drives a needle deep inside it. There is no way of preventing the pain of the procedure because it is the essence of pain itself. Needles in the legs and arms. And once inside the nerve, inside the white blindness of feeling, he asks me to move the limb attached to that nerve. And then it's the kind of pain that makes my body wish for blackout.

I get up from the table and my clothes cling to me with sweat.

Running

My younger sister Kate gets married in March. It's the most beautiful wedding I've ever attended. I wear a brace under my sock to keep my foot upright. On the second day of festivities I get a text to say my film, *The Sound of People*, has won the Belfast Film Festival.

I dance for the last time.

Bergerac. We go on holidays with my parents and my older sister's family.

No one is talking about my foot but we all know something is coming. It's like a deliberate holiday into innocence.

Ruth is under a lot of pressure. It's the not knowing: it's a weight, a silence between us. And yet we don't want to know.

We play games as best we can.

We're sitting on the grass and I get a call to say my film has won the grand jury prize in the Festival Opalciné in Paris and that on the jury is the iconic French actor Dominique Pinon. I lie back in the grass.

One day it rains and I carry Jack between the two houses. I pick him up and run through the rain. He clings to my body as the rain patters loudly through the trees. The fragile boundary between strength and weakness, between holding Jack and letting him fall: I feel it. The last time. And time slows down. I'm running in my sandals across soft earth and leaves, focusing all my energy on not letting go of Jack. There is no one else around. He trusts me completely. We run beneath the trees. We make it to the house.

He tells me

We cross the glacier at midnight. A row of bobbing head-torches in a sea of darkness. Ice-axe, crampons and a pipe over my shoulder for water. And more stars than I thought possible. This is outer space. We climb through the night.

The sun is up and I see where I am. I'm twenty thousand feet up a Himalayan mountain, lying on a four-foot-wide bridge of snow and ice that leads to the summit. We are an hour from the peak and I have never felt more tired in my life. I try to move. There is a sheer drop on both sides. I freeze. What am I doing here? And then I feel it. Immediate and sickening in my stomach. The shocking starkness of it inside me. If I fall here, I fall to my death. There is no one here to help me. I am alone. With it comes a feeling I have never felt before. I've thought about it many times but never felt it. Death. My death. It is as close to me as the drop on either side. It is all around my ears. I have to move. I start to climb.

I'm in his office and he tells me. Light leaves the room. And air. And sound. And time. I sit on the chair opposite but I am far away. Deep inside. Looking up through a tunnel of myself, as he speaks on past those words. 'Three to four years to live.' I don't hear him. Is this my life? Is he talking about me? I leave the room, the tunnel all around me, and stand before my wife in the waiting room. The colour leaves her face. Her father is beside her. They come into the room and he tells them the same thing. I don't hear him. Ruth starts to cry. Within ten minutes we are out on the street. Not knowing what to do, we do what we had planned to do before. We go to lunch. Ruth's dad will meet us after.

We walk through the streets like the survivors of some vast impact. Pale, powdered ghosts. We reach the restaurant. Dunne and Crescenzi on South Frederick Street. Our favourite. I stand into a doorway outside and call my parents. It is the worst phone call of my life. I tell them everything, fast, hearing the panic in my voice. Later, I'll thank them for coming when they arrive at our house, and they'll look at me as if I'm insane and I'll become aware, for the first time, that nothing is the same. We enter the restaurant. Sit down like everyone else. We sit there, not knowing what to do, what to say. The waiter comes over and starts to speak to me. Ruth starts to cry. The place is under water and I can't hear what he's saying. Ruth is pregnant with our third child.

We are orphans of the universe. Our species is defined by asking questions, out into the dark, without anyone to guide us except each other.

Time is a trick. From an outside vantage point we live a certain length of time, one that we measure in minutes, hours and seconds, birthdays and anniversaries. But we don't live at a vantage point to ourselves: we are immersed. We live in fits and starts and jumps, like dreams. And the lives we inhabit are measured in moments, irrespective of time. How we live is strange and uncertain and not written on any map.

In a movie, when a doctor tells a patient they have a certain time left to live, it sparks a voyage of discovery, a quest for authenticity and redemption. In *Joe Versus the Volcano*, one of my favourites, Joe Banks, when told he has a 'brain cloud', goes outside and hugs a large dog, then goes on to do what he's wanted to be doing for years: he lives his life.

I think of him often in those first days after. How that moment I had always laughed at had become my life. What now? What do I do? And it comes to me very quickly. I suddenly know what is different between me and Joe Banks, between all the stories and my life. I am happy. I am exactly where I want to be, doing exactly what I want to be doing, with exactly who I want to be with. It's quite a realisation to discover beyond doubt that you're happy. And death had brought me there.

Death. On my shoulder. In my head. In the garden. At the door of my office. In every glance with my wife. My new companion: the end of my life.

We are living in North Cottage, with our two little boys, Jack and Raife. We moved here so we could afford to live the life we wanted to live. I was working on my films, Ruth was writing her first novel and the boys had a garden ten times the size of the one at our previous house. We had a plan. And it was working. We were happy.

But that was before. This is after. Never before had I felt that split, but now a fault line has opened between our past and present, and there is no going back. Death, which before had lived on some distant horizon, is now in our living room. We are lost, within the familiar surroundings of our lives. Ruth and I cry a lot, at night, in bed.

Human time is not measured by clocks and watches. Time slows down, time speeds up and the mystery of how we live is ever present, despite our will for it to be otherwise. Our lives are not the legacy we leave behind, or the value of the work that we do. Our lives happen in between the deeds and ideas that define us. Each of us feels it, the mystery, the strangeness of life on earth. Of life and death. We feel it when we travel, we feel it when we stay at home. We feel it when a loved one dies or when a loved one is born. I'm sure we all crave more certainty than we have but that is not human life. That is the ticking of a clock.

When you are told you will die within a certain period, time slows down. Life becomes dominated by the last time. Is this the last time I will read a book to one of my boys? If not the last, how many more? How many? Everything is heightened. I stand outside in the darkness and watch my son playing in the window of the cottage. I stand until the cold is in my bones and wonder, Is this the last time that I'll stand? I'm in my life and outside it, in the moment and conscious of the significance of every moment.

It's lucky. In this heightened state, experience is burned into my memory. I'm running after Raife and I'm thinking, Is this the last time I'll be running? So I speed up. I'm running with a limp, and so running full tilt becomes a series of long hops and strides. But I'm running, across the grass, after my son, who is laughing uncontrollably, in the half-fright ecstasy of pursuit. And I'm remembering it. Fear of the last time is recording every second. Which is lucky, because it is the last time. And when you lose something central in your life it's important to have a memory of it, so you don't feel insane, so the pain you feel has a corresponding shape, something that says definitively, 'That was real.' Then, happy or sad about it, I have that for ever.

The hopeful and the desperate

I and my family are determined to prove the diagnosis wrong or find a treatment. So we pursue every thread. Every possible mimicking illness, every alternative blood test, every experimental trial. It is a long road, but it gives us hope, a focal point to lift our eyes from the life that lies in tatters all around us. Because that's the thing about your death, and the threat of your death: it's not just about you, it pulls in all your loved ones. Everybody's life has stopped.

I pursue treatment with everything I have. I'm not going to die like this. This isn't my life. I visit healers up and down the country, down bumpy side roads to mobile homes on breeze blocks, where the hopeful and the desperate sit outside in their cars looking self-consciously into the drizzle, waiting for their turn to step into the musty blend of Catholicism and mysticism, and the exchange of cash for hands that heal and a strange typed bit of paper with further instructions involving home remedies and prayer.

Ruth and I drive up to Letterkenny to see a healer my mother has found. We see him in a hotel. Queue up with others in the hall. A mother with a young son. A man. Inside the room the healer has stuck up yellowing news clippings all over the wall and the TV plays a scratchy documentary from an old VHS. All attest to the healing powers of this man. All show a much younger man.

A nice old gent, he performs his jiggery-pokery, touching my head with holy water, and we leave, no worse off, and have lunch in a little vegetarian café on the hill.

Ruth and I love weirdness: it's a part of who we are, the sense of humour we share. We seek it out, in life, in movies and books, that unique tilt on things that just tickles us. And this is grade-A weirdness. But we don't laugh. We don't talk about the truth of it. We're searching for hope and we're desperate.

The healer says it's better if I see him again (scam), and Ruth and I are more than happy to drive on to Galway for the next appointment in a day's time. We book into the hotel where he will be and go out for dinner with my sister and her husband, Kate and Pierre-Yves, who live there. It's a holiday.

In the morning I get the lift upstairs and find the room where the healer is staying. He does his routine and I give him money, thank him and leave. He brings a mustiness to the room and a loneliness. Travelling around like a broken bit of Ireland, a suitcase full of dogma, as desperate for belief as the people who come to see him.

I do reiki three times a week with an accountant outside Drogheda. She does part-time sessions out of her home. I have a second-hand convertible Golf and I drive with the top down through the long roads of trees by the water three times a week. It is amazing. It is so good, in fact, that I find myself thinking that I would not be without these experiences, that I would not choose otherwise. I come out after a session and the world is alive and green and full of hope. It is a start.

I read books about people who had cured themselves of cancers the size of basketballs, of how sickness is repressed emotion expressing itself on a cellular level. And in all the books the same refrain: you are the cause, you are the cure. I determine immediately that if I am in any way causing this I must take it on. I start seeing a psychiatrist.

Old-school Freudian, lying on my back, the psychiatrist sitting behind me in the half-darkness with a notepad and pen. I go for it, give it everything I have, determined to uncover any emotionally damaging activity. I mortify myself. Probe every private and emotionally embarrassing corner of my mind and speak it aloud in the hope that it will do some good. Fear of death leaves me fearless of anything else. I raise the roof.

I go once a week but the going is slow. Too slow. I push myself to talk, to let it all out in the hope of a *Good Will Hunting* breakthrough. But it doesn't work. It is good but I can't escape my voice. So I quit. My psychiatrist doesn't take it very well. Apparently I am the first person ever to leave and she isn't very happy. I told her that I felt it was moving too slowly, that I needed something that would work a bit quicker. I told her it wasn't her it was me. What I really wanted to say was that if I had ten years I'm sure it would work fine but I didn't.

I go to the house of a woman who does a course based on one of the books I'd read. It's called *The Journey*. The author claims to have healed herself of a tumour the size of a basketball. I felt embarrassed in the bookshop buying it, maybe because I doubt a lot of these books, but out of all the books it spoke to me.

The house is a bungalow in the forest. I sit in her living room and she puts a blanket over my lap. I close my eyes, listening to the sound of her voice. Within a few minutes I am crying, then sobbing. Moments from my past crystallise before me, moments of hurt, of humiliation, of despair, and all the time her voice, pushing me to go on, go deeper. When I was a child I made myself walk into a pitch-black field because I was so afraid. I went into the darkness and found a field full of stars. And so I sit in this woman's armchair and cry like a child and afterwards she gives me soup.

In the driveway as I get into my car, she stands in the doorway and says, You watch those doctors' faces now, when they do their tests and see.

I had done it. I had freed myself of any damaging emotion.

At reiki the following day my lady puts her hands on me and says, What did you do?

I am on fire.

The result of all this is that, emotionally and spiritually, I am about the healthiest person with ALS you are ever likely to meet. But to the progression of the disease it does nothing. It progresses, does its own thing, works on its own timeline.

Arden

I have a bad limp now. Everything is in the shadow of my health. And yet we live. It is a shadow, a foreboding. Physically nothing really has changed except I have a limp. And everything has changed.

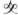

I work on the studio. I have men in to brick up the garage door, to plaster, to put the bathroom in. I'm buying the cinema gear from Richer Sounds in Belfast, the nicest guys you're ever likely to deal with. I'm in among the builders' cables and machinery measuring for speakers. Mathematics has never been my thing, but I'm in the studio at night, on my hands and knees, drawing chalk lines on the floor, working out the exact triangulation between the sitting position and the screen. The reason children sit so close to the TV is so the screen fills their peripheral vision and is totally immersive. Same principle. It is a labour of love.

I'm stepping among the coils of wires and men with my measuring tape when the voice of the contractor sounds beside me: That's an awful limp you have there.

I'm embarrassed. In the heat of the moment I'd forgotten I'm limping like Quasimodo. I hurt my back, I mumble.

⁂

I get the call. I drive beyond all reason through the city. It's the middle of the night. I find a space in the car park of the Coombe Hospital. I brace myself and get out of the car. The distance across the car park is longer than I'd thought. I look at the building ahead, at the metal railing of the walkway. I can make it. I have to make it. I cannot fall. If I fall I may not be able to get back up. Ruth is up there.

I make it. I'm sweating. People are looking at me, the smokers outside, as I cling to the rail, moving up the ramp to the double doors of the entrance. I have to let go. Another distance from the door to the elevator. Jesus. I move. My leg feels weak beneath me. I'm sweating heavily now. I see the guard behind the desk in front of me. I know if he stops me I won't make it. He's looking at me. I walk past him, dragging my foot into steps, my eyes locked on the lift door.

I make it. I make it down the corridor to Ruth's room. I brace myself, try to wipe the sweat and the crazed look from my face. I go in. Ruth smiles in the breathlessness of a contraction. I sit in a chair beside the bed, take her hand, smile. I feel like I've climbed a mountain.

Arden is born. A perfect, beautiful little boy. A war baby, Ruth and I call him.

I hold him on the couch and give him his bottle.

My brother-in-law's father, Claude, is a master craftsman. His work is in the Louvre. I admired a bookcase he had done for my sister's home in Galway, and he offered to do the same for us in North Cottage. Our books were sitting in boxes and there was a perfect wall in the living room. He arrives in a truck from Brittany.

Claude and his wife Véronique know of my diagnosis, and their response is in their eyes, heartache, love, despair. I love these people. Claude is a magical creature. His eyes are dark caves of light. Difficult to look into. Easy to get lost. He is here to work. I had expected shelves of some sort. What came out of his truck was eighteenth-century wood from the library of a château in Brittany.

For four days I watch them work. Father and son, Claude and Pierre-Yves. Now I knew why Pierre-Yves had been calling down for months, taking detailed dimensions and complaining about the complexity of the mathematical equations his father required. Claude had been preparing the wood for weeks in his workshop in France. Now I watch as they fit it to the space, creating something organic with this wood from far away that has always been there. This is wood as architecture, a structure of the simplest beauty. An art.

Claude will not accept money. So I give him a case of Guinness and Ruth gives Véronique Irish pottery we like. We are standing in our kitchen, all sharing a bottle of wine to celebrate the completion of the bookcase, when my legs give way. I collapse onto the tile floor. Everyone jumps, reaches out. I quickly haul myself up on the counter. It brings up the unspoken in everyone's eyes. But it remains there, unsaid, and we struggle back into trying to enjoy the moment.

Long after they're gone, I sit at night with the bookcase. Aged wood filled with all the books Ruth and I have collected over our lives. It makes me feel calm.

࿊

Ruth and I grow more haunted by the day.

I fall. I have been making myself walk up and down the hall with a walker twice a day. Fighting to stay on my feet. And one day I fall, badly. My body folds beneath me, my back bending to meet my legs. Our hall is tiled and I must have made quite a noise because Ruth comes running. When I see her face I know it is bad. I never walk after that.

🙥

I finish the studio. Put a wall of bookshelves and a desk under the window looking out to the garden. It's perfect. I have a red carpet put in and a local company builds a nine-foot couch. When it comes in the door it just keeps coming and coming. I import the screen from Japan. It's a third of the price of a flat-screen TV. It arrives in a box and my brother-in-law and I put it up. It's nine feet long and six feet high. The studio is finished.

It becomes a place for Ruth and me. When the children are asleep, we come out from the cottage to this adult space. I'm in a wheelchair we bought from Argos and we have ramps around the cottage leading down to the studio. In the dark, in the evening, we come outside, Ruth helps me out of the chair and we sit on the ridiculously long couch and watch a film in our private cinema. We invite friends and family and have Indian food and music before a movie. It is a happy place for us.

I wheel into this space I have created, slide across into my office chair and sit at the desk under the window. The smell of this room. The boys are playing in the garden. I start writing my new film.

But ALS does not let you rest. It does not let you adapt. It does not give you space. ALS takes and keeps taking. Or, rather, I keep losing more and more of my life. Every time Ruth and I take a moment to breathe, we are knocked back by this relentless ebbing death. And doom. The sense that all our dreams have already died.

This is what living with ALS is like. The battle between life and death. While I attempt to have a life, to build a life, it takes parts of me away. Death is a part of life and with ALS I am in a state of mourning. I mourn the loss of my legs and all that takes from my life. And my family mourns. But there is no resting. Never any resting.

My family is a force, a power of people. They rally. They find a clinic in England that is offering experimental treatment for ALS. I go over with my mum and sister Kate, who leaves her new husband alone to dedicate her time to me. We rent a little house by a forest in the snow. Dad is working in Ukraine. He flies here instead of home. I miss my wife, my children. After a month they come to join us in this quaint little house in the woods. A house called hope.

It's weird all living together. But it is my mum's chance to mother me in the face of this catastrophe. To feed me. To be a mother to her sick son.

Dad comes and we all eat dinner together. We watch game shows in the evening and play cards. We are a family.

The clinic is a strange place, run like a hospital but completely unapproved by conventional medicine. It is, again, populated by the desperate and the hopeful, I among them. Heavy use of intravenous antibiotics is the treatment of preference. It is a clinic born of market demand. Every conceivable alternative treatment is available. At a price.

We are all trying to believe it's not another scam. The most elaborate of them. It is my family's biggest effort. This has to work.

It doesn't.

I am getting worse and, after a while, we pack up and go home.

I hit rock bottom. We are trapped in North Cottage, our little house in the middle of nowhere, and every day it seems to grow smaller as our despair grows larger. Ruth, the boys and I are trapped in this fog that seems to permeate everything, to confound every effort. In the end, it is Ruth who saves us. Despite my fears and those of my family, Ruth takes us off to Australia. My family and I are locked in the fear of change. Ruth is not. She tells me we are going or we will go mad in this house. I believe her. I trust her. We go. Ruth, the two boys, our baby and me in the wheelchair.

Sunshine in our lives

They bring me onto the flight first. The plane is empty. They put me in this freaky contraption that strains the definition of chair, though it's called an aisle seat. It's a wheelchair the exact width of the aisle, which is bloody small. Two men lift me into it and wheel me down the aisle. They lift me into my seat and take the contraption away. I'm quite comfortable.

We take up the row, the two boys between Ruth and me, and Arden in a cot on the wall in front of Ruth. He is huge, he barely fits. Going to the loo on this long-haul flight involves peeing discreetly under a blanket into a bottle.

No one notices. Luckily I don't have to go to the bathroom as that would involve the dreaded aisle seat. Ruth has her hands full between minding Arden and ferrying the boys to and from the toilet. A woman across from me stares me out of it for just sitting there, the archetypal patriarch, while Ruth does all the running around. I sip my drink.

When the flight lands they come and lift me out of the seat. The woman comes over and says, Sorry, I didn't know. That's ok, I tell her. You have beautiful children, she says, and nearly runs from the plane.

Sunshine in our lives. We go for six weeks and stay for six months. It is one of the best times of our lives and it changes everything. Two of our closest friends are there and they adapt their lives to make ours easier. We rent a house with a swimming-pool, and start writing full time again, me for the Irish Film Board, Ruth on her novel. We see a psychotherapist once a week, a lovely woman who talks with you face to face, and we go to the cinema and eat a lot of good food. We are happy.

I realise that I have a simple choice: I can accept that I have ALS or I can give up. I realise that I have been carrying around the burden of responsibility for having ALS. That I was the cause but, through some failing of my own, I was not the cure. I had experienced first-hand the benefits of new-age therapy but, like so many systems of belief, genuine origins can often turn to dogmatic pronouncements of panacea. They can condescend to the sick, who are desperate to believe that the power to be better is within their grasp. But it is an unfair responsibility. People get sick. I wish that all things happened for a reason and that all things are in my power to change, but I don't believe it. And it's arrogance and a burden to tell someone who's sick that it's their fault if it's not.

❧

At the weekends we go to a café called Voyage, right down by the sea, with our friends Daragh and Cath and their son Theo. It does the nicest breakfast I've ever tasted, involving poached eggs, avocado and feta cheese. And good coffee.

Lifting the coffee to my lips, I feel, with sickening familiarity, the seesaw balance of strength and weakness. The question mark of whether I can hold the cup or let it fall. My arms. I try to hide it. But Ruth sees and feels everything.

We haven't outrun our problems but it feels like we're keeping pace here. Life is just too good to be buried for long. We go on outings with the kids, to museums, railways. Even the pleasure of the simplest playground is amplified by the weather. Days in the pool. At night we go to a cinema in a small forest, the roof a sea of stars. My friends haven't seen my latest short film, and I think, What if I could screen it here? So I send it into the cinema office and the next day get a call to say that they agree. It plays as part of an arts festival, and a journalist interviews me in front of the cinema crowd. It's my first time speaking in public from a wheelchair. It goes fine and my film plays among the trees.

We bring the boys to the lovely library up the road. We go to the ballet. We get a sixteen-year-old babysitter we can trust and Ruth and I go out for regular meals and to the cinema alone. What can I say? Australia.

ALS still lives in our lives. Every time Ruth helps me in the shower. Or we fight out of sadness and frustration. But the simple truth is that a better life helps all of us.

Pizza

I am getting weaker.

I'm sitting in the jeep in the darkness. The light from the pizza parlour is a white box with people inside. I see Ruth, her back against the window, sitting on a bench, reading a magazine. Jack and Raife dance around her seat, press their hands on the glass and stare into the fridge of chilled cans.

I cannot leave the car. I cannot walk. And it's too much hassle to use the sliding board to get into the chair just to pick up the pizza. So I sit in the darkness.

There is a restaurant adjoining the pizza joint. A very beautiful restaurant, which is why we come here for the pizza. It is dark and wooded and full of little lights. Men in crisp shirts smile as they enter with ladies brown from all day at the beach. Two older men sit in the outside section, facing the sea, their glasses of wine bright and clear in the evening light. Girls in white shirts move among the tables.

I watch the people as they enter. Their faces. Something on their faces. And then I realise. It's on everyone's face here. In the restaurant. In the pizza place.

Ease. Simple human ease.

It's evening, and between the stresses and strains, loss and pains, these people have found momentary reprieve. I don't know any of these people, but it's written on their faces. Something I have lost.

I have been told I am going to die. Very soon. And ease has left me.

Love. It's all it's ever been about. No one's story is more important than anyone else's. And only one thing scares me. Distance. From Ruth.

From my children. Daily distance. And death. The real distance. I can imagine it easily. Life without me. Ruth's loneliness. It's not difficult. It's easy. The stark strangeness of this life.

How to reconcile myself with my death. With my children standing by my bedside, crying, attempting to say goodbye. I do not know when that day will come.

I am not brave in the face of death. I am terrified.

Ruth said that surviving itself is a bravery. I don't know. I don't think I'm brave at all. Or that I handle my suffering with dignity and selflessness, as the books say. I try, and sometimes I succeed and sometimes I fail. Sometimes ALS buries me until I cannot see. Or if I do, I look out of a turtle shell and see a gaunt reflection looking back.

Other times, I touch what I once held. Arden asleep on my chest. Jack holding my hand in my wheelchair while we walk. Raife sitting on my lap. Ruth across a table from me in a restaurant.

Or being alone. Having pushed myself out of the house, down to the sea. Sitting under dusty palms, the wind in my face.

In Voyage, the awning flapping in the breeze. Sitting after breakfast over coffee and working on my film in my little notebook. Blissfully alone.

Time to leave

We go back. At Dublin airport both our families are there. We go into the bar before heading our separate ways. Everyone is jubilant, happy that our trip was a success, happy to see us. Our parents' faces are worn with worry. I lift my arm to shake hands with Ruth's dad and everyone notices the strain, the weakness. Everyone notices but no one sees.

We have a blissful summer in North Cottage. I now have an electric wheelchair as I no longer have the strength to push the manual one. I race around the garden with the boys. Through the apple trees. Along the path behind the herb garden. The sun is beating down and we play games for hours. In the evening we watch films in the studio. I introduce my boys to my love of cinema, as my father passed his to me.

We have decided to move. As much as we love North Cottage, the more ALS progresses, the more living in isolation becomes difficult. This wasn't part of our plan. A simple thing like driving down the road becomes a burden because I'm thrown around like a rag doll on the Irish country roads. Australia has shown us the benefits of living close to everything, to friends. Jack is about to start school. It's time to choose. Time to leave.

Fear

I get pneumonia in September. It's the first sign that ALS is affecting my breathing. Most people with ALS die of respiratory failure. I spend a week in hospital.

We're living in my parents' house while we look for a home in Greystones. There is a For Sale sign in front of North Cottage.

I take Jack or Raife out for spins in my power chair to Greystones town. It's a sudden independence. One at a time I take them on my lap, and we leave my parents' house, alone, just the two of us. We call it going on an adventure.

We go to the sea, the bookshop, the library, the supermarket but, above all, the video shop. It is our favourite place.

We take the back road from the house, a road from my childhood. Quiet, bumpy, full of memory. It's the quietness that matters, the solitude for me and my boy. The chance to be a father.

The weight of him on my lap. The shared silence of experience. The road. The trees. The half-hidden house we talk about. Then other people. We navigate. I cross the road like someone who is above the law. Abusing people's kindness, pity, fear. I don't know what they're thinking in their cars. I used to. I don't now. I'm different. And death is my VIP card. People stay back so I might as well play it. So I cross the road and everyone stops. Listens. Sees. I feel the weight of thought all around me. Some people thinking about me, others doing everything they can not to think. A man in a wheelchair with his son. So we cross, me and my boy, visible, invisible.

This is life in Greystones, the freedom to do things alone. In the video shop I can't reach up to the counter so Jack or Raife stands on my lap and pays the man. One movie for me and one for them.

We find a house in Greystones. It just feels right. We move a few doors, a wall. Home. We experiment with names but in the end stick with the number. It's a quiet little estate filled with children and you can see the sea from the back garden. Jack starts in a local school that my sisters attended.

North Cottage is sold. We have to say goodbye. To our library. To the studio. To the trees. It's not easy. We have lived here. I have to include all the cinema equipment to close the deal. They want the cinema. That makes me happy. Before we leave, I watch *Blade Runner* in the studio with my friend Phil. We turn the volume up to nine. It is sublime.

My breathing is getting worse. My voice has fallen to a whisper. We go for a family portrait in Dalkey with my family, my parents and my sisters' families. They lift me out of my power chair into a seat for the photograph. No one wants to see a wheelchair in the photo. Including me, I suppose. To everyone else it symbolises sickness. But when you are using a wheelchair, the negative symbolism is quickly replaced by the fact that this device is empowering you. My wheelchair is my friend. But this family portrait is about everyone else's point of view. And I am not immune. No one wants to see sickness. This is a portrait of the other parts of us. So we use another human symbol to represent our values. We smile.

In the pub after the photograph is taken, no one can hear my voice above the crowd. They lean in close but cannot hear.

I get pneumonia again. A double pneumonia, they say. I go into the Beacon Hospital. Ruth sleeps on the couch in my room. I'm terrified. I can hardly breathe and don't sleep for three days.

It escalates. We call the nurse. I tell him I cannot breathe. He looks at a monitor. Your stats are fine, he says. I cannot breathe. He just looks at me. I have twelve other patients, he says, and makes to leave. My brother-in-law, Chris, who is in the room, says, If Simon says he can't breathe, he can't breathe. He is six foot three. The nurse looks up at him.

I'm moved to Intensive Care. I can't breathe. I feel sheer panic now. I can't breathe, I tell the two nurses in the room.

They don't turn from the monitors high up on the wall at which they're staring. Your stats are fine, one of them says.

I'm drowning. I turn to Ruth, who is kneeling on the bed, one hand behind me, one in front, pumping my chest like an old squeezebox, helping me breathe. Don't stop, I say, raw panic in my voice. She meets my eyes and we share a moment of perfect fear. Ruth, help me, I say, and see utter helplessness in her eyes. She pumps my chest. Help me, I say, and the world tilts.

My country

You're in a room in Dublin. A man walks in whom you've never met. He starts to talk to you. He asks you if you have any children. You say you do. He tells you not to go home tonight. That when you leave the building you must turn right instead of left, head north instead of south. That you must keep going in an unknown direction, knowing only that you will never see anyone from your life again.

The journey he is asking you to take is death.

I come from a different country from you. A different place. There are only a few of us there.

My norm is very different from yours. You find it difficult to understand me. And, looking at me, you must think me quite strange. I have ALS.

I am in a bed in the Beacon Hospital. I went into respiratory failure, collapsed unconscious and was put on a ventilator.

I now have a tube up my nose and a tube down my throat. One for feeding, one for breathing. Both of which prevent me speaking. ALS prevents me moving my arms and legs. I communicate with my family through text messages on my phone.

A man has just walked in the door. I have never met him before and he starts to speak to me. He says his name is John Magner, consultant anaesthetist for the ICU. He tells me he has just got off the phone from Professor Orla Hardiman in Beaumont Hospital, after I requested that he ring them to ensure that I was getting the best care for ALS at the Beacon. He tells me that Professor Hardiman has said that they do not advocate ventilation in this country for ALS patients. That it is time for me to make the hard choice. He tells me that there have been only two cases of home ventilation but in both cases the people were extremely wealthy. Ruth and my mother start crying in the corner of the room. I look at him but I cannot reply. He looks at me.

Ruth and Mum are now holding each other, sobbing.

While he is looking at me, my life force, my soul, the part of me that feels like every part, is unequivocal. I want to live. It infuses my whole body to such an extent that I feel no fear in the face of this man. We find out two days later that the home ventilator is covered by the medical card.

❧

A day later, my father and I are watching a movie on my laptop. Every movie watched after talking to that man feels like a vindication to me. Every moment lived is a moment lived. We are watching the movie and another man walks in the door whom I have never met. He introduces himself as Ronan Walsh, neurologist. He begins to ask me about the history of my

ALS, despite my inability to speak due to the tubes. My father attempts to fill him in (medical details would not be his strong point). The man quickly gets down to the point. Why would you want to ventilate? he says. You have ALS and you are only going to get worse. At the moment you have use of your hands but the paralysis will grow, will get worse. Why would you want to ventilate?

For these people the questions *Why would you want to ventilate? Why would you want to live, having ALS, not being able to move your arms and your legs?* are rhetorical. But the irony is that they are asking the right questions.

Why would you want to ventilate? Why would you want to live? I have many reasons, if they are prepared to listen. But that is not why they are there. They are there because they have made a decision about my standard of living. To them it is inconceivable that I would want to live. But not for me. For me, it's not about *how long* you live but about *how* you live.

They ask me why I want to live and the answer is the same as that given by 'mostly dead' Westley in *The Princess Bride*, when replying to the question posed by Miracle Max: 'What's so important? What you got here that's worth living for?'

'Truue loove' is his response. That's how I feel. Love for my wife. Love for my children. My friends, my family. Love for life in general. My love is undimmed, unbowed, unbroken. I want to live. Is that wrong? What gives a life meaning? What constitutes a meaningful life? What gives one life more value than another? Surely only the individual can hope to grasp the meaning of his or her life. If not asked if they want the choice to live, it negates that meaning.

You have ALS: why would you want to live? ALS is a killer. But so is life. Everybody dies. But just because you will die at some point in the future, does that mean you should kill yourself now? For me, they were asking me to commit suicide. Or to endorse euthanasia. I refused. For days they stood around, scratching their heads and wondering what to do with me. In Ireland ALS patients are not routinely ventilated. They are sedated, counselled, eased into death. They are not given a choice. Not like in other countries, including the US. Not here. I was put on a ventilator in an emergency situation because the Beacon simply responded to my respiratory failure and saved my life. If I had been somewhere else, I might have been allowed to die. Imagine it. Something is deeply wrong here. I'm alive by mistake. They gave me my life and I wouldn't give it up. I believe everyone should be given that choice.

⁂

I am in the hospital over Christmas. During a snowstorm that stopped Ireland. I have got to know all the nurses. One girl, Bridget, from Cork, is pure heart. She walks across the road to the pub, buys a pint of Guinness and carries it back without spilling a drop. It's New Year's Eve, I think. I'm not sure. I'm on a lot of morphine. I manage a few sips of the Guinness. Another morning she comes into my room with a lunch box full of freshly fallen snow. Gently, she lifts my hand into the cool iciness.

✀

I take it. I don't need it. I want it.

I take the morphine. I have no pain. I don't take it for pain. I take it until Clint Eastwood's *Heartbreak Ridge* becomes a love story. I take it because it feels good. I take it and I love everyone.

The next day I cry for no reason. I take it again. I take it until a canny nurse cops on.

I take it until the line is taken out.

✀

We crave happiness. We are desperate for happiness. Advertising shows us epiphany after epiphany but we can't live up to that. We want to. We want to feel that in our lives. No one is exempt.

I am jealous. Of the movement of bodies like a drug. What is happiness anyway? I knew it once. The balance of elements tipped in one direction. I know it now in moments struggling to let myself be happy. It's difficult, when the elements are tipped the other way. Happiness is a moment above water.

Listen to me because I'm drowning.

I'm not a part of the world outside. The news doesn't talk to me. The weather is different light in the corridor. I wake up exhausted from a dream. Of running, of fighting on a bridge. What to do? To force myself awake. To summon all the effort just to move.

I've lost one sense and another is going. Smell is gone. I'm breathing through my neck now, not my nose. Taste is next. I've been eating boiled eggs for breakfast but that is becoming harder and harder.

I have a random urge for a Big Mac meal even though I'm vegetarian. It's bizarre. I mention it to my friend Kevin. The next day he arrives with a Big Mac meal without the meat. He takes out two veggie burgers, wrapped in tin foil, which he cooked at home, and puts them in the burger. I take bites of my veggie Big Mac, with fries and a strawberry milkshake. Taste.

My mum brings me in delicious home-cooked meals but a few choking episodes put an end to that. I no longer eat with my mouth, but by a small tube in my stomach, with nutritionally designed liquid foods.

Two senses gone. Three remain. I feel the slightest touch anywhere on my body.

Touch me. I see you. I hear you.

What have I become? To my children? I am still their father, always their father. But so different from everyone else. Everyone is different but some are more different than others. I feel for them, being in places where everybody's body works. Rooms full of people whose bodies work.

My family visit every day. Either they are visiting or they are minding my children so Ruth can come in. Or both. I cry every time my boys come in.

My sister Ruth dedicates all her time to getting me home. Kate knows every ALS website on the planet. My uncle Bobby arrives weekly with armfuls of films. My parents are exhausted.

My friend Phil visits me almost every day. He is a bedrock to me in this white world.

I don't know. I feel different today. Happy. It is a different feeling from anything else. Last night I dreamed I turned into the wind and flew. Round and round in cirrus spirals. So high it was beyond height. I woke up and felt like a king.

The days. They are our lives. I've forgotten what it is like to be the person I was. Those days. Sometimes it's so simple. I look at my father and see the same forces throughout his life. Family and his work. In that order. For ever. I'm that simple. We're cut from the same cloth. He has the soul of a cowboy.

I have been in this hospital now for four months and I am going home on a home ventilator. I am one of the first people with ALS to go home ventilated in Ireland with the support of the HSE. The HSE seems to get nothing but bad press yet they have been exemplary in their support of my move home. The nurses in the Beacon have been inspirational, guiding me through the terror of respiratory failure and the panic of recovery. I have been educated here in the vocation of caring. And the Irish Motor Neurone Disease Association has been unendingly supportive. For those two consultants, who, I have no doubt, believed that they were doing the right thing, believed that they were delivering the hard truth, I have nothing against them. But I do wish they would open their eyes. There is no hard truth, only truth on a given day by a given person. It is people who are hard or soft. And for every moment of hardness there has been an equal moment of kindness from a nurse or a different doctor, and I had many. A moment of kindness to a panicked, terrified patient, to the most vulnerable of people, allows the part of me that feels like every part to take a breath.

A consultant anaesthetist, Silvio Gligor, whom I have got to know over the long days here, comes into the room. He wants to say goodbye as I am going home in two days' time. He stands there, wrestling with his emotions, clearly wanting to say something of meaning to me, not just platitudes or farewells. The silence hangs about him as he tries to work out what it is. It is an emotional moment, rarely found between two men. When he finally does speak, this is what he says: Go home and teach your children many things.

I do not speak for all people with ALS. I speak only for myself. Perhaps others would question whether or not to ventilate. But I believe in being given the choice, not encouraged to follow the status quo.

Change is possible. John Magner, the consultant who told me I would have to switch off the ventilator, came in to see me after four months and told me I had come a long way and that he had learned a lot.

I am not a tragedy. I neither want nor need pity. I am full of hope. The word *hope* and ALS do not go together in this country. Hope is not about looking for a cure to a disease. Hope is a way of living. We often think we are entitled to a long and fruitful Coca-Cola life. But life is a privilege, not a right. I feel privileged to be alive. That's hope.

It's not important that you know everything about where I come from. About who I am. It's not important you know everything about ALS, about the specifics of the disease, about what it's like to have it. It's only important that you remember that behind every disease is a person. Remember that and you have everything you need to travel through my country.

A life

The nurses are crying. This is the goodness of people. They have come out with me in the ambulance home and they are crying because they are saying goodbye after four months together. I'm crying, of course. Four months is a long time in a room with no windows. They leave and I'm home. In my bed. In my bedroom. I can't take it in. It's all wood and colour where my world has been white. It's like butterscotch to my eyes. An orgy to my senses. I take it in.

I recover, but everything is changed once more. My hands are very weak. I use my touch phone as a mouse for my laptop so I can write. My voice is low and difficult to understand but I can still speak. I'm on a ventilator. The biggest change of all. The defining change. I now have a little box beside me that generates my breath, fills my lungs with the air my weakened muscles can no longer provide.

That little box has saved my life.

In the hospital I became aware that writing with my hands was becoming more and more difficult. An inspirational occupational therapist, Sarah Boyle, organises for a rep from a computer company, Nick Ward, to fly over from England to demonstrate an eye-gaze computer with me. It is extraordinary. A revelation to me. Freedom. My hands back, with the movement of my eyes.

Nick comes out to Greystones with my computer, funded by the incredible Irish Motor Neurone Disease Association. He is a gentleman with a droll British wit. He sets me up. A friendship is born. The computer enables everything: writing, internet, phone, text, TV.

I'm driving my chair with a switch operated by my head. Try and stop me.

Our lives have changed again. I now have a nurse day and night. A stranger in our home. Footsteps at night in the hall. But help, where before my wife and my family were struggling to survive. I no longer have to wake Ruth throughout the night. Independence during the day. Ruth starts to sleep, leave the house without fear. A life.

I watch an Irish documentary about ALS and am struck by an element at odds with my experience. It concerns Professor Orla Hardiman, head of ALS research and care in Ireland. In the documentary she is introduced as 'a tireless patient advocate'.

When I collapsed and blacked out in the Beacon Hospital, they put me on a ventilator to keep me alive. I woke up terrified and disoriented. When I gathered myself and realised the situation, my first thought was: I'm in the wrong hospital. I should be in Beaumont, under Orla Hardiman's care. But her response was: 'We do not advocate ventilation for patients with ALS.'

I and my family were beyond stunned. 'Do not advocate.'

My sister Ruth is a powerhouse and she gathers every piece of information about home ventilation and we forge our own path. But I think of those who don't have that support.

Ventilation and ALS is a sensitive topic. I write an article in the newspaper about my experience in hospital, and the paper gives Orla the right to reply.

In reply to my article, Orla and her team state that mechanical ventilation is discussed with all her patients, and that most don't want it (when they hear the details about it). She also points out that the resources simply aren't there to support ventilation for patients with ALS.

The other point she makes is that the problem for a person with ALS being on a ventilator is that it may be difficult for that person to communicate when they would like to come off the ventilator.

Communication is key with ALS because the disease takes your ability to speak. But it need not take your voice. Living in Ireland, with the support of extraordinary people, individuals with ALS can avail themselves of an incredible amount of technology that enables communication. Eyes, eyebrows, even the twitch of a muscle, can be utilised to give you back your voice. And while ALS can strip you of all such means of communication (the 'locked-in' state), though it's rare, this takes time, and you can communicate your wishes in terms of ventilation before that occurs.

To me, advocating for patients means fighting on their behalf, for their wishes.

Life on a ventilator with ALS isn't something everyone with ALS would choose. But for those of us who choose that life, I believe we need real advocates to support our choice.

Christmas

I start to write full time again with my eyes, using my new computer, as I start to recover, as my body grows stronger every day out of hospital.

I'm working on my feature script, and my sister Kate comes over in the afternoons and we talk about scenes. I print out drafts and poor Ruth knows the script verbatim.

We are struggling with the new routine, the constant presence of strangers.

My hands have stopped moving. My voice has become unintelligible. A slurring mockery of what it was. I use my computer voice for the first time, nervously, self-consciously. It quickly becomes my voice.

The principal of Jack's school asks me to write the nativity play for the Christmas Carol Mass in the local church. I accept, of course, and it becomes a strangely fulfilling task. The story of birth and love.

I have ALS. It is a part of who I am, evolving, influencing and living with all the other parts of me. The greatest achievement of my life is that somehow I managed to be the person that Ruth fell in love with. That's it. And our boys save our lives every day.

It's now four years that I've had ALS. The prognosis of three to four years to live did not factor in the ventilator. I'm past the four years and back out into the unknown, just where I want to be.

It's cold and autumn is turning into winter. The leaves move across the road, bright with the sun. We visited my parents today. My mother lit the fire in the kitchen and we talked of Christmas. And for the first time since I've had ALS I felt it. A fluttering, an anticipation, a dream of childhood Christmas. When we leave, the sun is shining and my soul is shining, like the winter sun.

Society is predicated on the idea that we all have the same wants and needs. But that's only when you reduce us to the same. What's different about us is just as important. The mystery of each of us. When we've read all the books our parents read, and missed a few, and read a few they never read, we still won't know what that person sitting opposite us on the train is thinking, feeling, remembering or dreaming. Never. Not for sure. Isn't it wonderful?

I'm sitting in a café. I have a pipe over my shoulder for air. The place is full of people sitting in twos and threes, talking over lunch. Two girls sit opposite me, leaning in across the table, deep in conversation. What are they talking about? I look around. What is anyone talking about in this sea of voices?

Truth does not endure. If it did, a great silence would hang over the earth. We take what we can from the past and make the rest up between us as we go along. It's wonderful. It means, at any given moment, anything is possible. Ruth walks back towards our table, carrying our coffee. She is pregnant with our fourth child. And our fifth.

The love of my life is pregnant. We are alive.

My willy works. It's that simple.

The day I found out that ALS didn't affect my penis was a red-letter day. Unlike a spinal injury or condition, ALS does not take away any feeling from my body. It removes my ability to send messages to my muscles to move. But as the penis is not a muscle, it is unaffected.

Other things remain. My eyes. Some of my facial muscles. I can still move a tiny muscle in my left hand. Just a twitch. But Ruth and the boys like to hold my hand while I move it, ever so slightly. It is a physical connection, however small. Raife calls it my imping.

Ruth and I treasure the physical connection we still have. And we had decided, privately, to try for another child. The ultimate expression of being alive.

We go into Holles Street Hospital for our first scan. Jack was born here, in the basement, six years ago. He came out blue and big. I will never forget. People's feet passing in the window. My first born.

We are in the room, the midwife, Ruth and I. Ruth's stomach being rubbed with jelly and the ultrasound. So you know it's twins, she says. You're joking, Ruth says. The woman looks a bit put out, as if the idea that she would joke while doing her job offends her. No, she says. Ruth and I look at each other, eyes wide, incredulous.

No, we didn't know, Ruth says. She and I are screaming inside. Would you like to know the sex? Yes. I think I say it through my computer or it might have been Ruth or I might just have thought it. Well, twin number one is a girl. Ruth and I start crying.

Ruth is gloriously big. Rest-a-cup-of-tea-on-her-bump big. It's cold. It's Christmas. We go down for the Carol Mass. I'm all wrapped up. As we move in the darkness, the cold crispness, moving with the people towards the yellow light of the church, I realise I'm as far from hospital as I can possibly get. I've made it. Out.

I've written a number of short poems to tell the story of the nativity, interspersed with carols. Sitting there, in the coolness of the marble, as the children give life to the poems, I am truly happy.

This day

People are amazing. I'm in the back of the car. We're moving fast. Riding bumps like waves. My chair lifting off the floor. In the back with me is my friend Cait from Limerick. Crazy. Has me in stitches most of the time. In the front is my brother-in-law, Pierre-Yves. French. Crazy. Drives like a madman. But he's not driving today. He's on the phone to his mother, speaking in a rapid rush of French. It's her birthday. My mother is driving. Bray. Crazy. Drives like a madwoman. I'm on my way to the hospital. Ruth's Caesarean is taking place at twelve. It's twenty to twelve.

❧

I believe in birthdays. I count forwards now, not back. I look ahead at forty and think, Yes. Yes, please. When I hear someone's age I subtract mine from theirs. Sixty-seven. Thirty years more than me. Old people are the worst. Ninety-nine. Sixty years more. Jesus. I look at older people with awe. You did it.

It's easier looking back. Twenty-five. I've lived twelve years more. Yes.

Then I look at my children, six, four and three, and I see how much they've lived in their lives, how much they've become, and I say, Wake up, learn something. It's all there for the taking.

Quite often, people who haven't seen me in the last four or five years find it almost impossible to reconcile the difference in me over that time. I don't blame them. I often find it hard myself. One way, for me, is to think I'm in my fifth year of ALS. The Second World War was six.

I'm nervous. In my stomach. I've been on this road before but nothing changes. Pierre-Yves turns from the front, his phone still pressed to his ear, and says, Mum says, did you know that Caesarean got its name because Caesar was the first child to be born that way?

No, I didn't know that. He slips back into the silk of spoken French. Caesar, I think. Caesar was born that way. Ok. The nerves in my stomach ease a little. We're approaching Holles Street.

History. All around us. Buildings older than any of us. The news telling us what's important every day. Yet there is a more important history. The things we gather. The photographs we hang. The things we use. Our living memory. The wake we leave behind.

When Ruth and I were searching for our first home, we walked into a bungalow we could not afford. Other people were walking around the house, in and out of doors. It was inviting, old-fashioned but immediately warm. The kitchen presses were simple seventies and the window above the sink looked out onto a garden run round with flowering plants. People stood in the garden. Ruth went on out. I stood in the room alone. I opened a narrow press by the back door. On a little shelf was a pair of gardening gloves, fresh dark earth still crumbling on the fingertips. I am transfixed. Embarrassed. Suddenly aware of doing something wrong. Why did I open the press? I shouldn't be here. I close it quickly and hurry out after Ruth.

When we go to leave I ask the estate agent. Yes, he tells me, the owner only passed away last week, an older lady, living by herself. The family are hoping for a quick sale. He smiles. I want to run from the house.

❧

They are waiting for us at the doors of Holles Street. Whisk us upstairs. My amazing people dress me in surgical gown, hat. Time has stopped. I enter the room.

Ruth is on the table. The medical team are beyond amazing, ushering me in, helping me get into the best possible position beside Ruth (Ruth later tells me if I had moved back and forth once more she was going to kill me [I was nervous]). They start. Ruth holds my hand. I watch everything. Sadie comes out feet first, screaming, blue. Then Hunter, bum high in the air but silent. Ruth and I look at each other. They lay him beside Sadie and he lets out a roar. Ruth and I start to cry.

So much history. The days I've lived. The places that linger, the single moment that stays, like something from a book you once read. Glimpses that live within us. We are strange.

We want to know. But we don't. If we knew how the body worked, there would be no disease. If we knew the mind, no pain. But there is too much to talk about. More mystery than history.

I write in bits and pieces. Live in bits and pieces. People live in my mind. People I've touched. A coffee and a cigarette at a small wooden table, with a girl sitting next to me. Knowing and not knowing. Love.

Pathways. Taken. Followed. And we end up having lived.

Leaning against a car, on a sloped German

street. Waiting for someone. Cloud and sun. It's cold when it goes in. I look up, the warmth on my face. I see an approaching cloud. How long before I'm in shadow? I follow its path towards the sun. I catch myself. Close my eyes. Feel the warmth on my face.

⸎

My extraordinary wife. I wouldn't change ALS. Those two babies in my arms. Their warmth against me. Rising and falling with my breath. I wouldn't risk that for anything.

Eucharist means thanksgiving. That's how I feel. Thank you, Caesar. Thank you, all who watched over Ruth and Sadie and Hunter. I send out a thank-you. A beacon. Something. From as deep as you can go. To as far as you can reach. I will hold this day inside me for the rest of my life.

⸎

Six months now. Sadie and Hunter are fat beautiful balls of life, with hands that reach to touch my face. ALS fought back these last few months, leaving me in terrified panic, drowning for air.

Last week I bit the bullet and admitted myself into hospital for the first time since I left in March of last year.

It was St Vincent's Hospital in Dublin, and the week I spent there changed my mind about consultants. The warm, sincere individuals I encountered treated me with the dignity of being a person, not a disease.

I don't know how other people handle ALS but sometimes it lays me so low that I don't know how I will go on. I feel like I'm being tortured, a thousand little jabs, which on their own I don't notice but slowly over time they start to hurt, until suddenly I'm crying. They're tiny things I barely notice, little hurts I've grown used to. Someone I love not understanding me. One of the boys telling me about something I will never do again with them. The hundreds of urges that I have to do simple human things but cannot do, like sit on a couch with Jack and read a book and hold him, put my arm around him, tickle him. I think I'm doing fine, then realise I'm holding myself together with I don't know what. Something unbreakable that pain keeps trying to break.

And then my boys pass the doorway on their scooters. Dot. Dot. Dash. Or wander into the room in their pyjamas, in the middle of some elaborate world of lizards and kings, the youngest watching his brothers with silent eyes of glass. Or one simply stands in the doorway, looks at me and says, Hi, Dadda. And I remember.

And I write. Writing is my fighting.

Some days you can just see clearly. Our meaning, what we value, is the most private part of us. It may just define us. It shapes everything we do, everything we say, everything we feel, everything we dream. It's hidden, from others, from ourselves. There is no mirror to show us what we value. So often it is only revealed to us after the fact, in the long movie reel of memory. And when we see it, our heart stops, aching with recognition. It is a beautiful thing to see yourself.

I'm still alive.

On the way home from the hospital I see my reflection in my computer. I have a black strap across my head and a white one under my chin, a pipe coming out of my neck and going over my shoulder. I look like some crazy desert horseman racing along the dual carriageway.

I'm still alive. I seem to thrive on things trying to kill me. I'm still alive, you bastard.

When I die, don't say, Simon loved films, say, Simon had as much love in him as blood. That's all. I'm racing towards a bridge.

What is man?

I had a different life. Before this one. Before death stood beside me. My death.

There is nothing romantic about death. It is terror.

A life. Now glimpsed in photographs and memory, of Simon as he was. Walking, talking, eating, drinking. Breathing. Simon.

How much is left of him? How much spans the divide between Before and After? What is Man? How much can be taken away and what is left?

I had a different life.

The tree

I'm lying on my back on the floor. The carpet in my room is blue. I'm in love.

She is a blonde-haired girl whom everyone loves, though probably not as much as me. Her face does something to me. Her body.

The carpet is threadbare but I like the feel of it beneath my fingers. This is my room. I'm fourteen.

I started writing poetry a year ago. Somewhere to put my pain. The things I can't talk about. I have a friend to whom I show the poems. He reads poetry. He understands. I love him too. Look up to him. Want to be him. I tell him all my secrets. Like about this girl I love. He has the confidence to talk to her all the time, at school, when we're down in the park. She touches him when he makes her laugh. But he does not love her. I don't know who he loves. She does not know my name.

❧

I'm going to see her today. I know it. I put on the shirt I like best. There is an open day at her school and everyone is going. It's the middle of summer.

I cross the landing. My sister Kate is in her room, listening to music. She is an angel. She is ten. I look in as I pass. She has an altar on her mantelpiece to Mary. Statues of all shapes and sizes. I see her on her knees sometimes. She is afraid of infinity, of the idea that things go on for ever, of Heaven. She wakes up crying.

I pass the door that leads up to the two attic rooms on the third floor. One is my older sister Ruth's bedroom. I don't go up there. She smokes out of her bedroom window. She is eighteen. The other day she came down her stairs and wordlessly handed me a book. *The Pawn of Prophecy* by David Eddings. I read it in a day.

A few weeks ago Dad handed me a copy of *The Grapes of Wrath* by John Steinbeck and said, You have to read this. A week later he gave me Joseph Heller's *Catch-22*.

I hear the radio from the kitchen. Mum is in there. She and I are friends. Mum is the centre of the family, a nucleus around which we orbit.

In the hall I see the television is on in the family room. It's Saturday. Dad is watching a film.

Film is a religion in our house. You don't speak during a film. You watch a movie from beginning to end.

My father taught me to love film. As his father had loved it before him. Dad grew up in the golden age of cinema before television. He lived in the array of individual cinemas in Dublin. The first film I saw in the cinema was when we were living in Cork. *The Cat from Outer Space*. I was spellbound.

When I was six I watched *The Godfather* with Dad. He talked me through all of the relationships. How Sonny shouldn't have spoken outside the family. He cried when Marlon Brando says, 'Look how they massacred my boy.' My love of cinema began.

My dad's brother, my uncle Bobby, is another cinephile. He is a polymath and the only adult I know with the patience to sit for hours and discuss anything at all. He is a part of our family and a massive influence on my life.

I've had a wonderful, happy childhood. But I can't stay in the house for ever. I go out.

I walk across the road to the tree where the group of boys I hang around with congregate. They are not my friends. They are a group of boys who delight in the humiliation of others.

Bullying is another word for humiliation. I don't know why I hang around the tree with them. My desire to have friends outweighs the cost.

I pass under the shadow of the tree. Straight away the slagging starts. They have noticed that I've made an effort with my clothes. They notice everything. Anything different. Difference is the currency of humiliation. I am different. A little chubby. A boy with two sisters, taught to love. An easy target.

I don't know how they notice my shirt. They start to say her name, that of the girl I love. My friend must have told them. He sits in the branches of the tree saying nothing.

Last week we were all up in a building site, muddy after hours of rain. Someone throws a mudball at me. Within seconds the group is in a circle around me, pelting me with mud. I hold my hands up to my face. They are all laughing. My friend is just standing there. I think I see him throwing something. I'm not sure. When they stop I run home. I climb up the front of my house to my bedroom. As I'm stepping in through the window, my mother walks into my room. Seeing me, my face, my clothes, covered with drying mud, she makes noises and says words I cannot hear. I'm drenched in shame.

It's my birthday. The doorbell rings. My parents are out and it's just me and my gran in the house. I'm upstairs and I hear Gran opening the door. Voices. Laughter. I feel it in my stomach. I come into the hall. They are taking the piss out of my gran and I can see she's getting flustered. She has Alzheimer's. They know it. I take my gran gently by the arm, tell her it's ok. She looks at me with frightened eyes and goes back into the house. I step out into the group of boys on the doorstep, closing the door over behind me. One of them laughs. I slap him in the face. He punches me in the stomach. I go down. They are all bigger than me. They get me up, make peace, cajole me, ask me am I coming out on my birthday. There is nothing in their voices. I close the door and walk out of the house, up the road.

We walk for a bit, take a turn onto a smaller road. They form a circle around me and pound me with eggs. This was their plan. When they've finished, I push one of them, the leader, and say, I hate you. I mean it in my bones. He laughs in my face. I understand then that I mean nothing to him. My love or hate, nothing. And something changes in me. I walk home covered with egg and shell. It's my birthday.

Standing under the tree in the shirt I like, I see them all from a distance. My friend is not my friend. He is cowardly. And the others are not just cruel to me but to each other. They snipe and chide and belittle. It's their only means of expression. It's pathetic.

We go down to the school. Me and this group of boys. I know she will be there. We wander through the school. The corridors are packed with adults and children. We enter a classroom. It has another door at the other end. There is artwork covering one wall and we start to walk past it as she enters through the other door, moving towards us, among a group of girls. Straight away the slagging starts, all around my ears. I feel my face grow red. I see her. She is beautiful. Unearthly beauty. Coming towards me. Burning inside and out, the words of the boys around me become a dull throb. I don't care about them. I care about this girl.

Four pieces of paper

My poetry is no longer about sadness, it is about joy. Love. The world around me. I have woken up.

If, in the earlier stage of boyhood, physical prowess was the defining characteristic, it is not in this stage.

I am no longer chubby. Coming from a house of love and women, I know how to speak to girls. In the place of brute force I have developed a sense of humour. I leave them in the dust.

Girls. The reason for living. The place for all my love. Difference. Beauty. Girls.

The back of their neck. The way they stand with their feet together. Their bare feet. The way they move when they don't know they're being watched. A tilted hip. Grace. Their shape. The softness of their skin, their arm, their face.

Girls. Girls. Girls.

Girls with big teeth. Girls with small teeth. Girls with big boobs. Girls with small boobs. Long hair. Short hair. Bad skin. Good skin. Thin lips. Full lips. Tall girls. Fat girls. Short girls. Thin girls. I fell in love with them all.

We're in someone's house and the parents are out. Four guys, four girls. The girls go off to four different rooms in the house. Four pieces of paper sit on the coffee-table in front of us. I take one. It says 'Toilet'.

Great.

I stand in the hall outside the door of the toilet as the other boys move off to other rooms. I don't know who's in there. I open the door. It's a tiny room with literally just a toilet. Sitting on the lid is a girl with ivory skin and black hair, a fairy of a girl. I close the door behind me. We look at each other, her eyes wide and dark. I've never done this before, I say. Me neither, she says. I lean down and we kiss. Our mouths touch and our tongues in the gentlest flutter of movement. My body is alive to her touch. I stand and we look at each other but don't speak. I leave the room dizzy with it. My first kiss.

Miles from home, in another town. The middle of the night. Full moon. I lie on a hillside in the embrace of a poem, writing furiously. I'm in love with the world and question everything from the beginning. What is the moon? I write how it feels to me, a burning drop on the cusp of the veil of knowing, and I must swallow it whole. I lie back in the dew-dark grass and drink it in.

White bicycles

I work in a local video shop. Thousands of films for me to watch for free. I have a soft brown chair in my bedroom and a tiny TV, which I have hooked up to four massive speakers mounted in the four corners of the ceiling. Perfect. I watch a film every night after work.

This is a literary culture and the question has always been, what book changed your life? But it is a film that changes mine. I feel embarrassed it's not a book. But you don't choose what changes you.

It's Peter Weir's *Dead Poets Society*. It speaks directly to me. It speaks to me in every way possible. I pledge to dedicate myself to writing.

I go out with girls. Long brown hair. Long black hair. Girls who make small sounds when we kiss.

I fall in love with a girl who doesn't love me back. I'm going out with her friend. It's making me miserable. We go down the coast camping. A group of us. That night there is a storm that blows down all the tents with sheets of rain. We run down a cliff path to the beach, to a cave, for shelter. We are soaked. When the rain stops I go down the beach and sit by the sea. The girl I love follows me and sits beside me. We don't speak. The moon throws a glittering path across the sea.

We sleep in the cave. All of us, in a pile. I wake up in the dead of night, frozen to the bone, teeth chattering. I touch my sleeping bag. Everything is soaked through. The sea is close to the cave now.

In the morning we eat burgers from a van.

I ring home. My dad shouts down the phone.

What the hell are you playing at? He tells me my mother had woken him in the middle of the night very upset saying, Where is Simon? He said, Don't worry, and touched her arm, and her skin was icy cold. Her teeth were chattering. Dad wouldn't stop shouting until I told him about the storm and that I was all right.

A few days later, over the counter of the video shop, I decide to stop being miserable. I decide to stop being in love with the girl.

※

I make a real group of friends at school. People who care about each other. People who want to share their experience with each other. Friends.

We are all in the same English class. The teacher is a doctor of English, and is bored to the marrow of his bones teaching the same curriculum for decades. He is even bored speaking and gives out in slow-motion, drawing out the syllables of each word: Miiii-chael, he says, you look like soooome-thing a motorcycle threw up, to a student wearing a leather jacket in class. The result is a unique English learning experience. Because there is only one thing that he does like. Stories. Our stories. He likes us to write them, to read them out in class, to discuss them. It is more like a creative-writing class than anything else. It is my favourite class.

I discover Ridley Scott's *Blade Runner*. It immediately becomes my favourite film. I have an attraction to its world that I cannot explain. I watch it over and over in my room.

I go to University College Dublin to study English and philosophy. I'm in my first long-term relationship. I'm having sex for the first time. I fail the second year. I'm in Cape Cod, east-coast America, working as a chef for the summer, living with my girlfriend in a little cottage, when I get the results. I get a fright, quit my job and go to the local library every day to study. I fly home and pass my repeat exams in the summer. I graduate third year with honours.

I leave the country with my friends, for Nuremberg, Germany.

I work the night shift in the largest printing factory in Europe. It is a small city. The staff are given bicycles to get around. White bicycles. I try not to count the cars of the freight trains that pass endlessly outside. It puts you to sleep. It's conveyor-belt work. Watch-the-clock work. I make up poems in my head. On my break I stand outside and eat German bread and cheese. I look across the industrial night landscape. White smoke and lights for a thousand miles. Men at work for a thousand years.

Winter in Berlin

From this hilltop the blue of the sea is in every direction. The blue of a cloudless sky. I want to live here. In the utter silence of the heat. Santorini. Mykonos. Ios. We burn all day, drink all night. It's been a long dark summer in Germany.

I return home to graduate but Germany draws me back. I'm at the bus stop in Greystones, listening to music, waiting for the airport bus. The music is stirring and I'm excited. It feels like the beginning of something. Berlin. A face steps in front of mine. The blonde girl I loved when I was fourteen. I'd heard she'd been living in Australia. She says my name, kisses me on the cheek and is gone before I can take off my headphones. I swear my feet leave the ground.

I arrive early to the building. It's dilapidated, covered with plastic and scaffolding. Next door is a primary school. Quiet, too early for children. I enter the plastic and climb the ravaged staircase to the top floor. The building has no roof. The floorboards are caked in ice and snow. Men stand in the shadows, smoking. It's my first day on the building site. The crew are grizzled and unfriendly. We are waiting for the foreman. It's freezing. Winter in Berlin.

The foreman arrives, looks me over once and joins the other men, muttering in German and looking in my direction. No one here speaks English. I have pidgin German. The foreman calls me over and the crew disperses, forming a wide circle around the two of us. The foreman walks over to an iron girder on the floor and bends down, gripping it. He indicates that I do the same at my end. You're joking, I think, looking around at the crew. They stare back at me. Apparently not. I lean down and grip the girder. I make eye contact with the foreman and we lift. It is an impossible weight, like nothing I've felt before. We don't break eye contact as he guides us across the floor. The foreman's face has turned red and a thick vein has risen on his forehead. I can't take much more. We put it down. He comes over, pats me on the back. I've passed the test. The crew is around us, all smiles. I'm offered a cigarette. I don't smoke. We smoke.

My first job is to stand in front of a wall while a guy knocks it down from the other side. As the tip of the jackhammer appears through the wall, I gather the bricks it dislodges and put them in a wheelbarrow. That's it. It's nerve-racking, waiting for the hammer to appear and the rush to grab the bricks. When the barrow is full I have to wheel it across a wooden bridge that spans the footpath five storeys below and dump it into a tube that feeds into a giant wastage skip on the street.

My first wheelbarrow is full of bricks. It weighs a ton as I push it towards the narrow bridge. The snow is compacted on the bridge and the result is sheet ice. The wheel starts to wobble as I cross. I slow to a snail's pace. I'm sweating, even in this cold. I inch forward and the wheel slips, the wheelbarrow flips, falling to one side, the bricks tumbling out. I lunge forward, throw my body across the bricks, grabbing the sides, trying to right the falling wheelbarrow. Pain sears across my back. It's too heavy. I manage to contain the bricks with my arms but a single solitary brick goes over the edge, disappears from view. Time slows. I don't know if I shout out. I think I do. I scramble to the bar and look down. Five storeys below I see a little girl in a red coat, schoolbag on her back, standing stock still. She is staring at the brick embedded in the snow of the footpath two feet in front of her. I feel the blood leave my face. She looks up at me then, her small round face as pale as snow.

I walk into the flat I'm staying in, absolutely shattered from my first day's work. My friends are there. I sit down. I almost killed a girl today, I say, and try to explain. They don't seem to get it. I fall asleep on the couch.

I'm going out with a German girl from a city called Wuppertal. She is an artist and paints on large canvases in her room at the top of the house, where wide windows open out above the city. We go to the pub to meet her friends. Walking home afterwards, we pass a long thin building, its windows gaping black holes, some boarded up. I ask what it is. It's the old train station, she says. Where the Jews were taken.

Drama

I have been accepted into a master's degree course in Anglo-Irish literature and drama at University College Dublin. I'm very excited. The course has attracted people from all over the world. China, Japan, a few people from America, Italy, Spain, me and two others from Ireland. Twelve in total. It's ridiculously intimidating. To me, they all seem to know a hell of a lot already about the subject I am there to learn.

Each week someone has to present an essay to the class. The first presentation is given by an American student. It solidifies the intimidation I feel. He stands, surrounded by piles of books and papers, and speaks slowly and calmly, totally at ease with his subject. He strokes his goatee as he talks, and uses the words 'demonstrative', 'indicative', 'Apollonian' and 'Dionysian'. I'm sweating. What am I doing here? I'm in over my head. He is speaking English but I don't understand.

I find out later in the library that they're just adjectives, adjectives with lots of syllables.

My turn. I stand, gripping a few pieces of paper, and read at the speed of thought. I'd be surprised if anyone understands me. The lecturer says, Any questions? And I look around with daggers at each person. No questions so.

I get to know another American student, here on a Fulbright scholarship and hilarious. He walks up to me after class and asks me would I like to be assistant director in a play he is directing for the university's drama society. That is why I'm here. Drama. Yes.

I love it. All the details of back stage. Casting. Art design. Costume. Props. Everything. The director asks me to play a part. Not my plan but I do it.

We're in the library, by the photocopiers. My director friend asks me to write a sign announcing rehearsals. I start to write, and realise I don't know how to spell 'rehearsal'. I'm mortified. How did I come this far and not be able to spell? Clearly there are gaps in my education. I look over at him and he is busy doing something else. This is a library. I grab a nearby dictionary and get the spelling. He hasn't noticed or is pretending he hasn't to be polite. I vow never to be in that situation again.

We put on the play. It goes without a hitch and is received very well. I'm hooked. To behind the scenes, rather than out front.

I give my last presentation. I stand, surrounded by books and papers, and speak slowly and calmly, at ease with my subject.

It's over. A friend is starting university in Edinburgh and I decide to go with him.

The biggest, thickest, heaviest dictionary

I work as a dishwasher. In the canteen of a petroleum-jelly factory. It gives me time to read and write and think. I get the bus in the darkness before dawn and read as it takes me out of the city into the industrial zone. I read in the fifteen-minute morning break and the hour for lunch. No one disturbs me. I make notes in my little black book. As the heat from the bacon pan warms my loins, while it soaks and I scrub, I think about what I've read and know my pen, book and notebook sit just over there under the counter by the hatch for dirty dishes. I'm a good dishwasher. The ladies play cards on their break. Kafka. Beckett. Camus.

❧

I get my first pay cheque and buy the biggest, thickest, heaviest dictionary I can carry. It is my prized possession. My father bought the complete hardbound works of Hemingway from his first pay packet working on the Underground in London. I have them now. I sit on the couch reading Beckett's *Murphy*, the dictionary beside me. I look up a word, which leads to another. I am in love with the etymology of words. I read the dictionary half the time. I get lost in words, stories like an inner voice. I'm living lives I didn't know existed. I walk the streets. My friend and I find a little video shop where the films are categorised by director and actor. I watch Wim Wenders' *Wings of Desire* for the first time.

On a tiny TV in a damp flat in Edinburgh, I sit on the floor in front of the screen as my friend gives up on the film halfway through and leaves. I am riveted. Glued. I can't speak afterwards. That way after the rarest of films. I have never seen anything like it. *Wings of Desire* is the *Ulysses* of film. The flow. The humanity of it. A moment on a bridge, with a man after coming off his motorbike, his last thoughts.

When films reach the heights of *Wings of*

Desire, Paris, Texas, Badlands, Punch Drunk Love, Blade Runner, Rushmore, they give me everything an art form can give. The things that keep us most alive.

❧

I start my higher diploma in education to become a qualified secondary-school teacher. It is more for my family than out of any real desire. To get a real job. The head of the course says, in his opening speech, This will be the hardest year of your life. He is right.

I'm teaching English in a secondary school in the morning and going to college all afternoon. At night I have to prepare my classes. I quite often sleep in my clothes, falling onto bed.

❧

I go to America in the summer, to Martha's Vineyard. I love America. At the end of the summer of work, a few of us go travelling with the money we have made. All across America by train, the glass car looking out into the desert. San Francisco. San Diego. John Fante. Charles

Bukowski. Bukowski reading Fante. Raymond Carver writing about Bukowski. Coffee. Breakfast. I love America.

Mexico. Peru. Bolivia. I drink it in. I'm writing all the time.

My father has worked in Russia for over ten years. The company he's working for have just bought a cement plant in Ukraine and they need a teacher to teach the management English. I'm in.

Cold from the fridge

I can see the road through the floor of the car. A blur of snow, I try not to look. The Lada is tied together with string. There is a piece of string across the hole in the floor. This is post-Soviet poverty at seventy miles an hour. The driver's shoulders reach the roof and he has to scrunch his head down just to fit. He looks like Luca Brasi. His name is Anatoli. My father is asleep in the passenger seat. Old-school traveller. Anatoli is hunched over the steering-wheel, squinting into the windscreen. I see why Dad is asleep. The windscreen wipers are going faster than the car but to no purpose. Outside is a total whiteout. I lean forward for a better look. Nothing. No road.

No sky. Just headlights into white nothingness. It appears Anatoli is navigating by some inner sight. Or homing beacon. I close my eyes and pray.

My father is a ground-troops capitalist soldier. Or, put another way, a chartered accountant sent to strange places. He was one of the first people into Kazakhstan, Kyrgyzstan, Uzbekistan, after the fall of the Soviet Union. Sent in by the World Bank to teach farmers who before had produced ten thousand chickens a day, all of which were bought by the government, to open a shop, to sell to the locals the produce of the small allotment they now owned. The embryo of capitalism. He came into a town with the idea of millions on his shoulders. He gave classes in purchasing and sales, debit and credit, profit and loss. He was the hero of capitalism, the vanguard of democracy. But it was all for nothing. The Mafia moved in and took over everything.

Now, years after the fall, Dad has been put in charge of a cement plant in southern Ukraine, with the cornerstone of capitalism as his mission. Turn a profit.

Six hours south of Kiev. We make it alive. Anatoli drops us off at my new home. It's a tower block, in a landscape of tower blocks. The company owns the bottom floor of this one, divided into two-bed apartments. Dad and I share one. Most of the workers live in the tower blocks. Two thousand staff and their families. As we walk from the car to the entrance I feel eyes from above.

I don't care where we live, I'm just happy to be living with Dad. Gold dust. I put up movie posters on the walls and at night we watch films and drink Ukrainian beer cold from the fridge.

They have never had a teacher and they get the carpenters to build me a blackboard. It's green. I teach the management team every morning and meet Dad for lunch in his office. Long, echoing corridors and the office doors are doors within doors so no one can listen, with lights above the doorway telling you whether or not you can enter. This is Kafka. Beside Dad's office is a queue of people waiting to see the Ukrainian boss, now second in command. Some have been there for days. One is asleep. Some will never get in to see him. Dad leaves the door of his office permanently open. It infuriates the others.

Sometimes after work we go into the old town and sit in darkened pubs and drink cold beer with paprika crisps. We like each other's company.

We are invited to a wedding. We are put sitting beside the bride and groom. I have an interpreter to my right. She whispers in my ear, translating all the speeches. She tells me who is sitting opposite us at the table. That is the local judge, she says, and beside him is the head of the Mafia. There used to be three Mafia heads, but one opened the front door of his house and was blown across the street, and the other drove his car off the road. I look at him. Shaved, gleaming, tanned head, he is young. Built like a house. He is a boxer, she tells me, owns a gym in town. In a jet-black silk shirt, he is the archetypal hood. He is looking at me and I stop thinking. I want to look away but I can't, not this close. His eyes are like a shark's. There is no other way to describe them. They are dead yet they are looking at me. And I realise I've never looked in eyes like this. I feel it deep inside. Fear. I look away.

Dancing starts. He dances with his girlfriend, also in black, apart from a red flower on her dress and the bright red of her lipstick. They dance and they look like flamenco dancers. I look around. Every pair of eyes is on them.

I talk to a girl taller than me. I'm six foot. She is a lithe Ukrainian. She says she has to go and I offer to walk her home and she says yes. We go outside and step down into the darkness of the trees by the road. Two large figures step out from the trees, blocking our path. Apparently I'm not supposed to leave the wedding. Dad has told me they're all armed. I look over and see the giant Anatoli, standing with the other drivers by the cars. I smile and wave, indicating that I'm ok to go on. He looks at me and nods at the two and they step back. I walk her home and we talk. She has perfect English. We reach her block and she goes inside and I don't get the kiss I was hoping for.

I'm going mad in the apartment so I phone the interpreter and ask if she would mind taking me into town. There is a population of over a hundred thousand and the large square at the centre of the old town is buzzing. It's strange to be out with you, she says, as we walk across it. Why? I ask. Because everyone knows who you are.

I laugh at the idea. I realise she is not joking. I look around. Here, there, all around the square, everyone is looking.

Gecko

I leave Ukraine after a year. My students give me a painting of the old town. It's strange to be leaving.

I fly to France to meet some friends for a holiday before I return to Ireland. Five of us go kayaking in the Dordogne for five days. I've decided to take a break from love.

I kiss a girl in one of the campsites. She is a tour guide from England and has a tattoo of a gecko on her ankle. The next day my friends and I are on a train to San Sebastián and I spend the journey drawing a gecko on my stomach with a blue biro. I show everyone.

We have to change trains. Waiting in a dusty rural station, we are all sitting in the shade when a bright green gecko runs across the space in front of us and right up to me, stopping between my legs. Everyone laughs and one of the lads tries to grab it. It darts away.

We go out in San Sebastián and I kiss a girl from America who tells me about her granny. She turns around to order a drink. On her back is a tattoo of a gecko.

I go home. I am taking a break from love.

Then I meet a tall, slender girl named Ruth on a bridge.

I spent my whole life looking for Ruth.

I stay over in her house in Harold's Cross for the first time. In her bedroom, on the mantelpiece above the fireplace, I pick up a small wooden carving on a necklace and hold it up to Ruth. I hand-carved that in Thailand, Ruth says. It took me ages. It's a gecko.

I'm still man

I do not eat or drink or walk or talk the way you do. I don't breathe without a machine helping me day and night. I cannot move my arms or legs. And yet. I'm still man.

I've lost so much. And yet. I'm still here.

I feel everything. The slightest feather touch anywhere on my body. And my heart is alive. To meaning. To value. To love. Which is all it's ever been about.

I realise I have a choice. I can let this life crush me. Bearing down on me until I am dead. Or I can bear the weight. And live. There is no surviving. There is living and dying. There are no gates to this suffering. No liberator will come. I must decide.

To live or die.

No pain without love. No love without pain. We are not built for death. It does not sit well with us. It is not in us. We cannot grasp it. I cannot. The end of me. It is beyond fear. Beyond reason. Beyond us. Yet the universal question: Are you afraid of dying? And the ever-evolving answer we formulate throughout our lives, secretly hoping we will truly believe it. Death is not in us, despite what the scientists say. Yet death is as real as our reflection. As present. A presence that we must ponder, must endure. Until we die. And become that which we are not.

This life is the harshest of opposites: Death and Love. Anyone who says different has not met death.

This life is ours, and whether we want to keep it or let it go, there is no love without pain, no death without love.

I'm a good man. I see it now. I've been selfish and spoilt but I've also been the best this life has to offer. The people I've touched, everything I've ever tried to do or say. Love. This existence is good. The sun on the fence. The people I've touched. I'm worthy of my sons' love now. These are an old man's thoughts. My body is afraid of death and so am I. To leave this place. But I have lived.

I stand before the vast stillness of the sea. I get that feeling, like in front of the Grand Canyon. When nature becomes a presence. And it's Me and The World. There is a noise above the waves, a rhythmic chopping sound. A man in the water, swimming alone, his arms cutting the surface, one at a time. His wake only a dark stain behind him. Humans don't leave much of a wake. I close my eyes. I am living. I am alive.

Some days I wake up blank, empty. And I wait for the day to fill me. Other days I wake up full, from a dream. And those are the days I despair. Because remembering is not feeling, and dreaming is not remembering. Dreaming is reliving. And then I wake up. And I feel like an old man. Dreaming of youth and waking up old. Dreaming of love and waking up alone.

And one day I decided I had a choice. I could fill my days with nothing or I could try and live again.

It's not yet dark

Ruth wants me to be a novelist. An easier life. But I'm not a novelist. I'm a filmmaker. A writer and director. And once you find out what it is that moves and shakes you, you don't want to do or be anything else.

I finish the script. I start looking for a producer. I find two. The kind of people who almost make me believe in destiny again. Kathryn. Lesley. We start to work.

My babies, Sadie and Hunter, are a light in my life. Every day they fill me up, like a battery depleted. Just to see their faces. I'm hooked.

If I'd said yes to the doctors telling me to die three years ago, they wouldn't exist. They are life.

Every profession is inconvenient to ALS (except perhaps a novelist or a mathematician …). But we don't choose what moves us, what drives us. It chooses us. Just like ALS chose me. You are what you are. It's up to you what you choose to do about it.

Ruth and I struggle with this life of ours. We worry about each other, about our children. We have a different life from many, and it is isolating. The strangeness of it. We wake up often, in the middle of the afternoon, in the middle of some simple action, and think: How did this happen? How did our lives become like this? And there is a sadness with it and a memory of a different life, lighter, like a remembered dream. Then it's gone, and we slip back into the stream of now, where our children are. I like being alive.

So I'm a filmmaker with ALS. What a whopper. It's certainly never dull.

Unlike other filmmakers, I'm unencumbered with the worries and stresses of building a career out of the work I love. ALS aptly strips you of such worries, coming as it does with far more pressing demands.

What remains is desire. The simple, raw, unending desire to make a film. Not as a statement, not to prove I can, not out of ego and not out of sheer bull-headedness. Out of love. For film. For the process. For the work. For the why we do the things we are driven to do. Driven to exhaustion because just at that point is the perfection that we seek, the all we have to give, given to an art.

And then Ruth comes into the room, with the freshest face I've ever seen, and asks me to come outside, to sit with her, it's sunny, and, as always in those moments, I can't hear her voice, I'm looking at her hair, her face, trying to take her in, and I'd better get my ass outside.

When James Joyce finished *Finnegans Wake*, he sat on a park bench and said he felt like all the blood had drained from his brain. That's what I'm talking about.

I'm not James Joyce but I know what he's talking about.

So that is desire.

The film I desire to make is *My Name Is Emily*, a story of a sixteen-year-old girl. It's been living inside me for the past five years. Emily fascinates me. Because I believe in redemption. I believe in the power to take what life throws at you and slowly to come back, to take all you have and not be crushed to death by sadness and loss. This is a story of redemption. People are crushed every day by sadness and loss. This is not an attempt to say otherwise. This is just a story where that doesn't happen.

I want to make a beautiful Irish film. Beauty fascinates me. I think about it all the time. Some films break my heart, prove that you can reach for human beauty in film, show how young an art form it is; beauty is only starting to be explored. Living as we do surrounded by the manipulation of the image, advertising becoming more and more lyrical, bending beauty to the task of selling, the question of beauty becomes more relevant and pressing. I find myself asking, what is beauty in cinema? Do we find figures backlit by the sun beautiful because they relate to some innate form of beauty within us, an idea of happiness, or is it a cliché that has formed to which we are responding? And I always come back to those films that remind me beauty is possible, that cliché hasn't taken over yet. The films that touch me, move me, push me.

It's two o'clock. The news numbers the dead. I am at peace. My son is putting golf balls in the hall. Over and over. He is four. Arden. I wish I could text into his head my love for him. Buzz around his ears, whispering my love. This is ALS. This is why I cannot touch him, stand above him, draw him in. So I project my love out into the hall, out into his life, and hope he hears me. Little footsteps in the hall.

There is a certain sickness to always wanting a happy ending, if the desire for it is driven by a fear of seeing things as they are. Popular media is rife with that desire. But there is another impulse, much deeper than fear. The will to live. To live with the sadness, loss and love that is this life. To navigate it. To not give up. That is Emily's story. It is mine.

Tell me your secrets. In the deepest depths of night, whisper them to me. Tell me your desires, if you can. Tell me your fears. Tell me what you like to eat. And how you like to eat it. Tell me details, as if you're half awake, half asleep. We are humans. I'm listening. Tell me with your body. Tell me with your mouth. Tell me why you think it's worth living. Tell me something I can keep. Without thinking, tell me something in the shape of you. Your skin prickles in the breeze, tell me, I'm obsessed with you.

It's not yet dark. I can see a chink of light through the curtains to the gloaming outside. All my children and Ruth are asleep. I'm holding her hand. The house is quiet. Yesterday was my first day casting. I was in a theatre auditioning actors, directing. I made it back to work. In 2008 the diagnosis told me it would all be taken away. And I made it back to work.

Take that away. Try.

This life is a magical life. I wake up feeling blue and Ruth brings in Sadie, my now one-year-old girl, to sit on the bed beside me. Ruth lifts my hand to touch her face and Sadie points at me. They only stayed for a few moments but after they leave I am changed. She is concentrated will to live.

I go down for Arden's first day of school. The air is fresh and bright before the heat of the day. After we drop him to his class we go down to the coast. The sun on the sea is sparkling.

The darkness

Sadie and Hunter find me.

They sit beside me in bed or on my lap in my chair. We listen to music. She holds my hand. He touches my face. Nothing makes me happier in the world.

I'm burning with this life.

Ruth and I go to the Wexford opera festival. We try to go every year. Last year I missed it because I was ill. We have to book the tickets six months in advance. Every year I make it seems to mark another year alive. We go this year.

I wear my tuxedo. I don't remember when I bought it. Ruth wears a simple black dress and I feel that familiar pride at being in her company. My dad drives us down. It puts us both at ease. We arrive at the opera house, but as we make to go inside my wheelchair won't turn on. For the first time in three years it has broken down. Shit. It's twenty minutes to the start of the opera and I can't move an inch. I'm stuck. Ruth and Dad are frantically making phone calls but it's Sunday night. Men in tuxedos run from the theatre offering their help. Ruth pulls a lever under the chair and suddenly I'm able to be pushed manually. But I still won't move. The safety straps holding the chair to the car will not open with the angle of the chair and we cannot adjust the angle without turning it on. It's five to. I resign myself to going home.

But Ruth won't give up. Someone gets scissors. Ruth leans down into the dark and cuts the straps. I'm free. Hands pull and I freewheel backwards down the ramp onto the cobbled street. More hands, and Ruth is by my side pushing with the others, propelling me across the road. Through a blur of tuxedos and ladies looking, through doors that open before us, and suddenly I'm in the packed opera house, in my place, and the doors close behind me. We go to turn on my computer but someone has left it on in the bag and it's overheated and is broken. I have no voice.

Ruth is exhilarated after the mad dash in here. She is electrified, her face vibrant and alive. She whispers in my ear. It's a sign, she says, you're stripped back, no technology, it's just you and the music. It's just you and you're enough. I can understand you with your eyes. She kisses me. Jesus. I'm in love with this woman.

The lights go down and stay down as the orchestra plays its introduction. I'm in the dark with all these people, as alive as everyone else. I feel a part of humanity, just sitting in the audience, no technology, no one looking. The timbre of the live instruments fills my senses. In the darkness, it's just the music and me.

Reading Group Guide

Topics for Discussion

1. "It's not important that you know everything about where I come from. About who I am. It's not important you know everything about ALS, about the specifics of the disease, about what it's like to have it. It's only important that you remember that behind every disease is a person. Remember that and you have everything you need to travel through my country." (92) How do these "directions" from Simon affect how you think about him and his situation? How might they change how you interact with people who are ill?

2. "Society is predicated on the idea that we all have the same wants and needs. But that's only when you reduce us to the same. What's different about us is just as important." (100) Why does Simon think people's differences are so important? He writes about his discouragement with the health care system deciding what is right for all people with ALS. How does that frustration relate to this quote?

3. Alan Rickman said *It's Not Yet Dark* is "beautifully written" and "utterly life-affirming." Did you find this to be true? Given the subject matter, did you have any concerns or expectations for how you would feel reading the book? Were your expectations accurate?

4. What does Simon mean by "seeing yourself" on page 111? How do you think his lifestyle and having ALS might allow him to understand or see himself differently from others?

5. The idea of choice is so important in this book. On pages 151–152, Simon explains: "I can let this life crush me. Bearing down on me until I am dead. Or I can bear the weight . . . I must

decide. To live or die." On page 156, he says, "But we don't choose what moves us, what drives us. It chooses us. Just like ALS chose me . . . It's up to you what you choose to do about it." How has Simon's life affected how he considers his choices? Is his understanding of choice similar to your own?

6. On page 156, Simon describes the moments when he and Ruth realize the "strangeness" of their lives, but then any sadness passes, and they return to their new lives. What does this say about Simon and Ruth, and also about the resiliency of people to adapt in order to live?

7. "There is a certain sickness to always wanting a happy ending, if the desire for it is driven by a fear of seeing things as they are . . . But there is another impulse, much deeper than fear. The will to live . . . To not give up." (160) Do you agree with Simon? Is this specific to Simon's story? Is it a common story?

Conversation with
Simon Fitzmaurice and Sam Gillette, of People Magazine

from

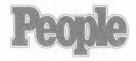

Award-winning filmmaker Simon Fitzmaurice was just thirty-three when he was diagnosed with ALS in 2008 — and told he had no more than four years to live.

His wife, Ruth, was pregnant with their third child at the time, but Fitzmaurice refused to bow down to despair.

In his memoir *It's Not Yet Dark,* which was released in the United States on Tuesday, the Irishman traces his journey from the tragic diagnosis (ALS is a progressive neurological disorder that is usually fatal) to reclaiming his life and work as film director. Fellow countryman Colin Farrell narrated a documentary of the same name, which highlights Fitzmaurice's inspirational story and opens in theaters on Friday.

"A beautiful love story—in its essence that's what this is," Farrell said in a blurb for the book. "Survival stories are not about surviving, they're inherently about what makes a survivor push through. A desire to remain in the light of all creation, even as a darkening is taking place. A darkening which happens to us all."

In an exclusive interview with *People,* Fitzmaurice shared details about his memoir and how he stayed in the light: through his work and his family, which now includes five children. Now confined to a wheelchair, he wrote his responses with an eye-gaze computer. This is the same device that allowed him to direct *My Name Is Emily,* which was released in the U.S. in February and won best cinematography in an Irish feature at the Galway Film Fleadh in 2015.

What is the biggest challenge you face while directing a film with your condition?

The biggest challenge in filmmaking that comes with ALS is time. When I'm on set, there is a short delay while I type up my thoughts. I overcome this by preparing as much as possible in advance of the shoot. Preparation is key. I spend a very long time storyboarding, thus reducing unnecessary discussions on set. Storyboarding each shot, so that everyone involved knows exactly what we're doing all the time. Pre-production is seriously intense.

When it came to filming, it was like any film shoot, it is a frenzy of creativity and very long days. I barely saw my family for the six weeks. I would come in from a twelve- to fourteen-hour day and have to prepare for the following day. It is its own momentum. My sister, Ruth, was my rock. Every day she was there round the clock, standing by my shoulder . . .

ALS is defined by loss. By what it takes away. But this was me taking something back. I returned to work. And that was a great feeling. To be back on set. Because it's the work that I love.

Why did *My Name Is Emily* resonate with so many viewers?

The story of *My Name Is Emily* lived inside me for five years. Emily fascinated me. Because I believe in redemption. I believe in the power to take what life throws at you and to slowly come back, to take all you have and not be crushed to death by sadness and loss. This is a story of redemption. People are crushed every day by sadness and loss. This is not an attempt to say otherwise. This is just a story where that doesn't happen.

There is a certain sickness to always wanting a happy ending, [as] if the desire for it is driven by a fear of seeing things as they are. Popular media is rife with that desire. But there is another impulse, much deeper than fear. The will to live. To live with the sadness, loss, and love that is life. To navigate it. To not give up. That is Emily's story.

What inspires you as a filmmaker?

My writing usually comes from a key phrase or thought. Very often it will become the beginning of a story. In this case it was: Life happens quickly, like mountains in the background. And you wake up one day. And you don't know how you got there. I'm obsessed with the act of waking up. As a sudden, new awareness of yourself. A sudden new perspective of your existence that moments before didn't exist. It's a fascinating human phenomenon. Fascinating enough to me to weave a story out of it.

How has your family been impacted since your diagnosis?

Living with me isn't easy. I have noisy equipment, ventilators and beds that wheeze and whistle all day and night. And strangers come into our family home, nurses to help me live this life. They quickly move from strangers to familiar faces, but it is an unusual family environment. And all because of me. And all because of ALS. I worry all the time about the effect that I, and

ALS, have on my loved ones. The price of me being alive. It takes a lot of effort to facilitate my being alive. People are amazing. I simply know that it's worth it to me. I value my life. I value being alive. And I just hope I give back to everyone to make all the effort worthwhile. I'm in love with this life, and it's worth every hardship to me.

What do you want your children to take away from your memoir?

My wife asked me to write a letter to each of our children, a personal letter to each, saying how I felt about them, memories of our time together, an explanation [of] how ALS had changed things. Something they would have to keep when I die. It was the most difficult thing anyone had ever asked me to do. I tried for years. But every time I started a letter, I was immediately overcome by the act of saying goodbye for the last time, and I would get no more than a few lines before my screen dissolved into tears.

I didn't want to write the letters and yet

felt so guilty for failing to write them. I was afraid of writing a book because I was scared of touching again the pain of the previous years. But nothing frightened me more than those letters, so I started to write. The book quickly became a comfort to me. Every morning I would write a little, always busy with my film, and it became a time of quiet, comforting reflection. I went back and it was okay. It was a journey. But above all, for me my book is a letter to each of my children.

What would you like your readers to know?

To quote my book:

"Our lives are not the legacy we leave behind, or the value of the work that we do. Our lives happen in between the deeds and ideas that define us. Each of us feel it, the mystery, the strangeness of life on earth. Of life and death. We feel it when we travel, we feel it when we stay at home. We feel it when a loved one dies or when a loved one is born. I'm sure we all crave more certainty than we have but that is not human life. That is the ticking of a clock. Some days you can just see clearly. Our meaning, what we value, is the most private part of us. It may just define us. It shapes everything we do, everything we say, everything we feel, everything we dream. It's hidden, from others, from ourselves. There is no mirror to show us what we value. So often it is only revealed to us after the fact, in the long movie reel of memory. And when we see it, our heart stops, aching with recognition. It is a beautiful thing to see yourself."